Come Back Strong

BALANCED WELLNESS AFTER SURGICAL MENOPAUSE

Lori Ann King

Gunnison Press
KINGSTON, NY

Lori Ann King/Gunnison Press
Email: info@loriannking.com
Website: www.LoriAnnKing.com

Book Layout ©2018 BookDesignTemplates.com
Copy editing by Stephanie Gunning
Cover design by Gus Yoo

Ordering Information: Quantity sales. Special discounts are available on quantity purchases by corporations, associations, libraries, and others. For details, contact bulkorders@loriannking.com.

Library of Congress Control Number 2017916564

Come Back Strong/ Lori Ann King. —1st ed.

ISBN 978-0-9995423-0-9

This book is dedicated to women in all stages of hormonal transition who are seeking the peace and serenity that comes from balanced wellness.

Contents

Acknowledgments

When I sit down to write, it starts as a quiet, solitary journey, just me and God, probing my heart and experience to find stories from my personal experience that could inspire others to lead lives of true health, love, laughter, and freedom. Along the way, the team of collaborators grow, as more and more people show up to contribute their expertise, until finally, the finished project of my first book is in your hands. The following people were part of my creative circle that allowed *Come Back Strong* to come to fruition.

My heartfelt thanks to my husband, best friend, and playmate, Jim, who loves me in sickness, health, and menopause. Thank you for supporting, encouraging, and believing in me. Thank you for always pushing me to be a better storyteller. Thank you for calling me out as an author long before I had the courage to whisper my dream to become one. And thank you for your willingness to share the vulnerable parts of our lives so that we could inspire others.

Thank you to my sister, Kathy, for being the biggest cheerleader. I love our early morning phone calls. You inspire me to follow my dreams and live on purpose.

To my mom and dad, thank you for instilling in me a strong work ethic and a belief system that I could be, do, and have anything my heart desires. Thank you for your love and support through all the challenges and victories of life.

Thank you, Dr. Dean Bloch, for treating me with kindness and respect as we worked to balance my hormones and help me feel vibrant and healthy through surgical menopause.

Thank you, Carolyn Rabiner, for your guidance, support, and friendship. You always point me toward balanced wellness, reminding me my body, mind, and spirit know how to heal.

I thank my editor and publishing consultant, Stephanie Gunning, for her guidance and skill to help make my first book a reality.

To Gus Yoo, thank you for the production of the cover design.

Thank you, Ruth, my high school friend and fellow author. You encouraged me from the day you found out I was a writer. Thank you for your faith and support over the years, and for reading my work and offering honest feedback. You believed in me even before you read a word of my work.

Thank you to Susan Vitolo, for sticking with me as my friend and workout partner at times when I wasn't the best version of myself. Your faith and perseverance inspires me and I'm grateful for your friendship. Thank you for reading my early work and showing me where I'm writing from a place of anger and perhaps need to deal with that to write a better story.

Thank you, Holly, one of my newest friends. I loved you from the day we met. You give me a fresh perspective, always reminding me to include a few surprises and find ways to make serious subjects a little lighter. Thank you especially for homemade peanut butter banana fudgesicles on your front porch.

Thank you to the amazing friends, mentors, healers, guides, visitors, and early readers who have touched my life and believed in me. Thank you to Susan Sly, Camille Lawson, Mark DeCesare, Shari Ackerman, Theresa Lyn Widmann, Michelle Renar, Lori Pociask, Leslie Melvin, Karen Homan, Jocelyn Noelle Boettner, and Lori Hudspeth.

Thank you to Davene and Mark, for creating the Master Key Mastermind Alliance Course. Thank you, Nancy Ottinger and the entire MKMMA team, for your guidance in developing my definite major purpose, better habits, and believing with me in my dreams and in the power to manifest them.

Foreword
Carolyn Rabiner, L.Ac, Dipl. C.H.

WITH INTELLIGENCE AND PENETRATING INSIGHT, Lori Ann King has given women who are facing, or have already had a hysterectomy and/or oophorectomy, the gift of a much-needed guide to help with the fear and confusion that often accompany this experience. She accomplishes this with candor and humor, freely sharing her own personal experiences and feelings on numerous topics that are common to having these procedures, including many that women are hesitant to discuss with their friends or even their doctors. Lori's experience as a health and fitness coach really helps here. The reader will find numerous resources for finding her way back to wholeness.

Lori introduces readers to important new ways of thinking about the experience of hysterectomy and surgical menopause. She deeply explores the plethora of feelings associated with this, from beliefs a woman has held before discovering that she has a problem, and the shock of first learning about what is happening, all the way through the post-surgical phase and recovery Lori provides powerful tools, along with numerous suggestions for further learning, that will help readers to heal more quickly, and indeed, improve their lives in many positive ways.

Lori has a keen understanding of the mind-body component involved in the healing journey. With a clear and engaging style, she includes fascinating new research findings on this emerging science. Her many tips and ideas for how to deeply connect with this aspect of one's being will inspire readers to explore facets of themselves that can kindle healing and transformation. For the reader who is willing to be "captain of her own ship," the implications here are nothing less than profound. Arrival at a state as challenging as surgical menopause can be, can also be understood as an urgent call to dig deeply into one's being—to learn to trust one's own instincts. In this way, one can experience life-changing breakthroughs. For example, when Lori wasn't happy with her medication, and had reached a state of exasperation, she found an alternate route to complaining to her doctor. By applying the techniques she outlines in her book, her condition greatly improved, and subsequently she was able to find balance with a lower dose of bioidentical hormones.

This is only one of many triumphs that are detailed in these pages. Lori came back strong, and so can you!

Introduction

THIS IS NOT THE FIRST book I thought I'd write. It's not even the second or third that was on the list. The more I wrote, the more I released anger, anxiety, sadness, and overwhelm from my heart and body, and let in more light in the form of forgiveness, peace, joy, and ease. Writing was therapeutic. Almost two years after my hysterectomy, I was still seeking balance. So were other women. I continued to write and publish about my recovery while connecting with women from all over the world who were struggling just like me. My writing took a turn toward awareness, education, and empowerment for women everywhere. Writing became about doing service.

I'm not a doctor or a hormone specialist. I'm simply a woman who was having an ovarian cyst removed and woke up having had a hysterectomy and in full-onset surgical menopause.

This book explains what I wish I knew ahead of time and what I have since learned. I have heard other women say that they were "never the same" after hysterectomy. While I believe that's true, menopause can enhance who we are. It intensifies things that are out of balance. If a woman is struggling with her weight, finances, career, purpose, another illness, passion, focus, or drive, surgical menopause will make each of these issues more obvious and extreme. Surgical menopause will rush the symptoms to you all at once.

The foundation of this book is my personal experience and what I did to help myself. I had to recover from more than the removal of an organ and the tiny incisions the surgeon made in my abdomen. As I moved through this transitional time in my life, my body and mind transformed. My hormones changed and it felt like every aspect of my life was out of balance. I sought to heal old wounds and rediscover passions from childhood. It was a time of personal discovery and creative expression. I questioned who I was and who I wanted to be in the future. I found myself putting all areas of my life, from relationships to career, hobbies, and interests, under a microscope for examination.

The quality of my life improved with this surgery. I no longer fear unbearable pain, heavy periods, or endometriosis. There is relief in knowing that I am not at risk for diseases like ovarian cancer. This life event forced me to develop tools that could change my thoughts, words, and feelings so that I could live on purpose and with passion and clarity. Overall, I had a lot to learn. I still do.

How to Use This Book

If you are reading this, then you may be in one of several places in your life. Possibly:

- You're facing surgery, illness, or treatment that could push you into surgical menopause.
- You know a woman who is going through surgical menopause and want to learn the best way to help and support her.
- You are already in surgical menopause.
- You are going through natural menopause and looking for ways to improve your health and wellness and regain your balance.
- You have an interest in learning more about balancing yourself after medical trauma.

Regardless of where you are, within these pages are tools that can strengthen your mind, body, and emotions and assist you to live a more balanced life. Use them all or use a few. Above all, don't take my word on anything. Try things out for yourself.

If you are facing the possibility of surgical menopause, you'll want to read Chapter 2, "Preparing for Surgery and Initial Recovery."

If you already have a healthy diet and exercise routine or if you are struggling with anxiety and depression, focus on Chapter 6, "Thoughts, Words, and Feelings," specifically the section "Tools to Change Your Emotions."

If surgical menopause has shined a light on the fact that you lack passion and purpose in your life, then jump right to Chapter 7, "Come Back Strong."

I wrote this book for women who are preparing for surgery, as well as women who are facing what comes after it: surgical menopause. Despite the pain or struggle you are in right now, if any, this book was written to offer you hope that you can feel amazing despite surgical menopause. I'm living proof that it is possible, and if I can come back strong, you can.

CHAPTER 1

My Story

EVERY WOMAN WILL ONE day arrive in menopause; however, the intensity and duration of symptoms will vary. Surgical menopause is different than natural menopause in that it is often more abrupt, more intense, and depending on the age when it occurs, lasts longer. Here is how it happened for me.

A Woman of Strength

Strong. Empowered. Joyful. Confident. That's how many of my friends describe me. It is how I feel. It is who I am.

I have a natural curiosity and sense of adventure. As a child, I was always smiling, exploring, and clowning around. I was a tomboy, always wanting five more minutes to play outside. In high school, I was the class flirt and prom queen who went to college to study Recreation. In my twenties, while training for the Vermont City Marathon, I would rise at 5 AM to get in my mileage. After I got home, I would shower, eat, grab a cup of coffee, and head to work with a skip in my step. I'd arrive at my job ready to conquer the day, smiling cheerfully and asking everyone in my path, "Hey, did you catch that *brilliant* sunrise?!"

Yes, I was that woman.

I spent over two decades running and racing any distance from two to 26.2 miles. In my late thirties, I became an elite cyclist who excelled going uphill. Then, my inner athlete found a home in the gym, adding strength to my endurance. I learned to do my first pull-up and went on to succeed at doing over fifteen in a row.

In 2014, at age forty-three, I was in the best shape of my life. I was strong and lean at 119 pounds. I had the six-pack abs to prove the work I had done both in the gym and in the kitchen. That year, I participated in a sixteen-week transformation challenge that involved a before and after photo and an essay. Out of over 3,000 participants, I was proud to receive an honorable mention.

Around this time, I was due for a routine colonoscopy. This may seem young to you, but the test was appropriate because my mom is a colon cancer survivor and I had a history of digestive issues including constipation, abdominal pain, diverticulosis, and irritable bowel syndrome. I postponed the procedure for a few months until my "after" photos could be taken and my challenge was officially complete. I didn't want to take any unnecessary risks with what the prep, anesthesia, or recovery might do to my abs.

Hey, once you have them, you don't want to give them up.

Testing and Waiting

The procedure went well. However, my gastroenterologist ordered an ultrasound and a CT scan to see if anything was pushing on my intestines that might explain some of the pain I'd been experiencing. This led to the discovery of a small mass near my cervix and an ovarian cyst. I was referred to my regular gynecologist.

Now, when my routine test results came back, and they included the word *mass*, my blood pressure went up a notch. Cysts I knew were common and relatively harmless. I knew they could come and go on their own. I was pretty confident that a cyst would not kill me.

The idea of a *mass*, on the other hand, had a whole different connotation and stress factor. I admit that the possibility of cancer crossed my mind. I wish I had asked more questions. I might have heard that while it could be cancer, it could also have been a fibroid. We would not know until it was removed and tested. A fibroid sounded much more manageable than cancer in my mind. Language is powerful, as is the reassurance of an answer to a clarifying question.

Did I mention it was December and we were in the middle of the holiday season? My stress levels might have been higher than normal. This testing and waiting didn't help matters.

I made the call to set an appointment with my gynecologist. I was told he was booked solid for several months. When I explained my situation, they informed me I could get in sooner if I saw another doctor in the office.

In hindsight, I might have pushed a little harder to see my regular gynecologist with whom I had a seven-year history. However, in my rush to move forward quickly, get things taken care of, and get back to some form of normalcy, I opted to see the unfamiliar doctor.

My husband, Jim, came with me to this consultation and together with my new doctor, we decided to remove the mass and monitor the cyst. Just days after my colonoscopy, I was back in surgery to have the mass removed. More anesthesia. More recovery.

In the end, the mass was not cancer. It was a fibroid. Benign. I breathed a sigh of relief, took a few days' rest, enjoyed the holidays, and got excited for the New Year and getting back to living my healthy life.

Four weeks after the fibroid was removed, Jim and I traveled to Palm Springs, California, for a wellness conference. We left our hotel, had lunch, and walked to the convention center. By the time we got there, I was doubled over in pain. I was carried off on a stretcher and transported by ambulance to the local hospital. We spent our entire day at the local hospital where I underwent a battery of blood work, tests, and X-rays.

Can you imagine? Talk about embarrassing. My life and passions are built around health and wellness, and I was carted off on a stretcher from a wellness event.

Nothing was found, and the pain receded. Looking back, it may have been pain from endometriosis that had yet to be discovered. Endometriosis is a condition where tissue normally inside your uterus grows outside it and can cause pain, fatigue, and constipation. It could also have been an incidence of irritable bowel syndrome (IBS). I had gotten dehydrated, hadn't slept well, and had a high-fat meal at an unfamiliar restaurant. Also, my stress levels had continued to rise due to traveling. These are all variables that can lead to an IBS attack. IBS is a disorder that affects the large intestine (colon). Symptoms, which can include cramping, abdominal pain, and bloat, are very similar to the discomfort that can occur during a woman's reproductive cycle.

When we got home from our trip, I wanted life to go back to the way I knew it before this six-week battery of tests and procedures. I was sick of doctors and of being poked and prodded and tested. I wanted whatever was going on in my body to go away. Fast.

I went back to the gym. I enjoyed our indoor cycling workouts. I knew I was not done, that I would have to revisit the ovarian cyst, but I was not overly concerned. I thought the worst was behind me.

Three months after the discovery of the fibroid and cyst, an ultrasound revealed that the cyst had not gone away on its own as we had hoped.

In fact, it had grown.

I decided it was time to have it removed and be done with this once and for all. My new doctor told Jim and me that in the best-case scenario she would remove one ovary where the cyst was attached and its connecting fallopian tube (a partial *oophorectomy*). The actual outcome, however, depended on what she found. She informed me that the worst-case possibility was that I would require a full hysterectomy. We accepted the first available surgical appointment four weeks later.

Done. We had a plan. I wasn't worried. This was no big deal. I'd had a fibroid removed in December. It only took a week or two and my life was back to normal. When the doctor mentioned the worst-case scenario, I barely paid attention. I'd already had two procedures and recovered. I thought, *All is well. This will be fine. In and out procedure. Piece of cake.* I believed that the only difference between the best-case and worst-case scenarios was the amount of time it would take me to recover physically.

Did I say I wasn't worried? I lied. I was worried, although I was telling myself not to be. My body, however, knew that I was. And for the four weeks between deciding to have the ovary removed and the actual surgery to remove it, I was worried. And scared. And stressed.

It wasn't just that I had an ovarian cyst that wouldn't go away. Many women have ovarian cysts that are harmless, without symptoms, and go away on their own. But there is the possibility they can continue to grow large, twist, rupture, bleed, and become painful.

While I was nervous about signing up for a third surgical procedure in four months, I chose to have the cyst and ovary removed because of my lifestyle. I'm a cyclist. Jim and I will ride one hundred miles or more in a week into remote areas with sketchy cell phone service. The concern over the cyst and the possibility of a painful attack were reason enough for my decision. I'd also had a history of heavy bleeding: a three-week menstrual period, a few days off, then three weeks of heavier bleeding. That alone was exhausting. As an endurance athlete, needing a bathroom every hour had an inconvenient impact on life. Furthermore, I did not plan to have children.

I've Fallen and I Can't Get Up

On April 16, 2015, back into surgery I went, hoping and trusting for the best-case scenario: the simple removal of one ovary and its fallopian tube. I was excited to erase the pain that was burdening me. I didn't expect anything else to happen. My new doctor would be in communication with Jim throughout surgery and decisions would be made on my behalf while my only task was to remain unconscious and trust that I was in good hands.

I awoke to learn that the worst-case scenario had happened: I had received a full hysterectomy as well as a double oophorectomy. Uterus, cervix, ovaries, fallopian tubes—everything had been removed due to the severity of endometriosis that had been found.

I expected to be pain free when I woke. It didn't work that way. I was in severe pain. I was tired. I was afraid. I couldn't pee or poop. My body felt and looked swollen and bloated. This was uncharted territory and I had no idea how to fix it.

I spent one night in the hospital. I was on pain meds and my new doctor prescribed an Ambien to sedate me, to no avail. Sleep would not come. I awoke every hour or two, and in the morning felt exhausted. People were in and out of my room all night, often the reason I would wake up. Nurses had different tasks to perform. Some came to draw blood or check my temperature or vitals. Some, it seemed, simply came in to erase a name off the board and announce loudly that their shift was changing.

I had a history of panic attacks, and this was a breeding ground for anxiety. I cried at the drop of a hat for what seemed like no reason. My breathing sped up, my heart raced, a lump developed in my throat, and I felt the anxiousness that comes from a panic attack. As I tried to calm myself and slow my breathing, feelings of worry and depression would roll in. I no longer felt healthy and vibrant. I felt like I had fallen into a pit of darkness and despair. And I couldn't get up. How long would I feel this way?

Jim arrived in the morning to take me home. Although we were told I would be discharged early and quickly, somehow that translated into several hours of waiting. And crying. And anger. It was around this time that a nurse came into my room to check on me and innocently asked why I was crying.

"Because I just had a fucking hysterectomy!" I shouted at her, immediately embarrassed, but too frustrated to stop myself. If Jim could have crawled under the bed right then, he would have. I thought from embarrassment or shame. He later told me, he was just plain scared.

So was I. Who was this person that had taken control over my mouth, screaming and cursing at innocent caretakers? Was she even human?

Anger quickly turned to humiliation, guilt, remorse, and shame, partnered with a fresh new set of uncontrollable tears. Later, I apologized.

My new doctor who performed my surgery was not available to discharge me, so another doctor came to counsel me before we left.

I remember feeling uncomfortable and frustrated with the idea of yet another new doctor, but wanted to go home nonetheless. I was embarrassed at how quickly and ferociously I had snapped at the nurse who was simply doing her job and being kind. I didn't recognize myself or how I felt. I scared myself with my outburst. I felt ashamed for not asking more questions ahead of time to prepare myself. Questions about what this worst-case scenario meant for my recovery and the rest of my life. Was it too late to ask?

Embarrassed, scared, and ashamed, all I could think to ask this stranger was when I could return to work. He suggested two weeks. I remember thinking, *Two weeks sounds like a long time to start feeling better.* A few days later, a friend who works in the human resources of her company advised me that a hysterectomy is considered major surgery, meaning I was entitled to six weeks of short-term disability leave. She recommended I take at least that.

At my follow-up appointment the week after surgery, the doctor who performed the surgery agreed that this was indeed what was within my rights to take and advised me to accept the full six weeks if I could financially afford to. While I didn't want the healing process to take this long, I was grateful to have the time to rest and recover without the added stress of working.

Even in the twenty-first century, crying is not an acceptable practice on the job.

Fighting to Heal

It was at this first check-in that I was prescribed bioidentical hormone therapy (BHRT) and began applying daily creams of both estradiol and progesterone to my skin. I wanted desperately to heal and feel normal again and was willing to do anything to get suddenly well.

In the weeks while I was at home recovering, I found myself explaining and clarifying and justifying to family and friends. Conversations would go something like this:

Friend: "What's new? I haven't seen you in a while."

Me: "I had a hysterectomy."

Friend: "Oh. Wow. What else is new?"

Me: "No. I had a full hysterectomy."

Friend: "Okay. And?"

Me: "I had a full hysterectomy and oophorectomy. They took everything. Nothing's left of my womanly parts except my va-jay-jay."

Friend: "Oh. Okay. So that's simple these days, right? An in-and-out procedure? Laparoscopic? Barely a scar? When will you be back to work? Wait, why are you crying?"

This experience had turned my world upside down and it would feel as if my friend was saying "So what? What's the big deal?" The big deal was that I was struggling both physically and emotionally and I didn't know how to help myself feel better again. I didn't know how to regain my balance. I felt weak.

The reality was, after a few days, I was out and about. I went to a business meeting even though I felt awful. It hurt to walk, sit, and stand. I couldn't get comfortable. I had about an hour of energy to spare before I needed a nap. Yet people I spoke with months after that meeting had no idea that anything about me had not been normal. I felt I had to be strong and silent and push through.

Surgical menopause is a "silent" situation. Everything can look normal from the outside; meanwhile, nothing feels right or familiar on the inside. The physical pain subsides, but the crashing fatigue lingers.

At my six-week checkup, I was still feeling emotional and unstable and had lots of questions and symptoms I wanted to be addressed. I was referred to my original doctor, Dean Bloch, M.D., a local expert in BHRT.

I was relieved. Dr. Bloch had been my doctor for over seven years. He treated Jim and me as valuable members of my wellness team. He listened and addressed my symptoms and concerns, often suggesting outside reading to help me understand my options. I was grateful to be back with someone familiar who would partner with me in a holistic approach to my health.

Over the course of the next year, Dr. Bloch adjusted my hormone therapy. He increased the doses of estradiol and progesterone based on blood work as well as my reported symptoms, which eventually became complaints. These included hot flashes, night sweats, fatigue, insomnia, loss of libido, weight gain, lack of focus, zombie-like state, depression, anger, and overall lack of passion and energy for anything in life. At one point he added testosterone to my regimen.

I learned that hormone therapy is not an exact science. In fact, it seemed a bit like a guessing game as we attempted to balance my hormones and emotions and help me feel good again. The hardest part, perhaps, was that it simply took time to get it right.

My memory of thinking two weeks was a long time to heal would haunt me. One month. Six weeks. My mood swings and I returned to work full-time. I tried to hide in my office, yet I ran into people from my department who hadn't noticed I'd been absent for six weeks. They didn't know what I'd gone through or that I'd had surgery. But then, what did I expect? I'm a private person, and in a sense, I didn't want anyone to know what I was struggling with.

Or did I? I am human and at times, I do long for empathy. I want to feel significant. Good, bad, or ugly I want to be seen. The feeling of not being seen and my struggles not being acknowledged is probably the root of why conversations with friends and family made me cry. While I didn't expect anyone to "fix" me, I did long for compassion.

I had trouble talking about the surgery when I got back. I ran into a cycling friend who also happens to be a member of the executive board where I work. He asked if Jim and I had been doing much riding. Tears filled my eyes and the lump in my throat made it hard to explain that I hadn't been on my bike at all since having surgery.

Navigating the return to work was indeed hard after this kind of surgery, as it can be after any absence due to illness or the death of a loved one. Is there a protocol? Maybe a memo could have been sent out before my return. A warning, if you will.

> *Dear Coworker of Lori,*
>
> *We just want you to know that Lori had her insides ripped out of her six weeks ago. She will look normal on the outside. On the inside, she is in a state of confusion due to the sudden drop in hormones.*
>
> *No, she doesn't want to talk about it. No, she isn't tan from going to the beach. Please don't ask her if she enjoyed her vacation. Don't ask her anything because she may cry. Or yell. Or drop an F-bomb.*
>
> *Yes, you can bring her tea and tell her how much you missed her.*
>
> *Sincerely,*
> *Lori's Surgical Menopause Management Team*
>
> *P.S. Silent hugs are totally acceptable.*
> *P.P.S. Expect tears.*
> *P.P.P.S. And an occasional F-bomb.*

I found myself feeling lost and misunderstood as I navigated my journey through surgical menopause. Everything, from getting up in the morning to getting myself through my workday and finding the energy to socialize and maintain relationships, became laborious.

I felt alone because I didn't know anybody who had gone through exactly what I was. I felt misunderstood because even when I tried to explain what I was going through, people still didn't understand.

Two months. Three months. Six months. A year. A year of struggle when all I wanted was to ride my bike and feel good in my body again. A year of sadness and emotional turmoil where I would cry for no reason. I remembered being an outgoing, vibrant woman filled with joy. Now I was a listless crybaby. I'd lost my curiosity, zest for life, and drive.

I was frustrated with how I felt and how slow the healing process took. Symptoms of surgical menopause became a vicious cycle. I was prone to gaining weight, which made me feel depressed and unsexy, which led to a loss of libido. Night sweats kept me up at night, as did my thoughts of trying to figure out how to fix myself or lose weight. Insomnia led to fatigue, lack of focus, and a zombie-like state. I subsequently took in massive amounts of caffeine and sugar to get through the day, which resulted in highs and lows, energy crashes, and disruption to my sleep cycle.

And no matter how much I knew about nutrition and exercise, when I felt like crap, I ate like crap. Hence, I gained weight. Alas, the cycle continued. This was not easy to accept or admit. As a wellness and weight-loss coach, I'm supposed to know what to do. But this cycle of menopause symptoms affected every aspect of my life, including my confidence in my ability to lead a healthy and balanced lifestyle.

I was also angry. I was angry about this sudden condition that I didn't sign up for. I was angry for how awful I felt. I was angry at being angry. I whined, criticized, and blamed everyone and everything for my suffering. I blamed the surgery. I blamed my doctor. I blamed Jim. I blamed myself.

I eventually blamed BHRT. After sixteen months of attempting to compensate for my hormonal imbalance with BHRT, I still felt less than my best. I had given BHRT a good try and still felt like crap. I decided to try going the other way and weaned myself off BHRT completely. Many people, including some doctors, agreed with this decision, and predicted that I would begin to feel better right away and the excess weight I had put on would fall off me with ease.

Dr. Bloch, as patient as ever and always listening, accepted my decision and reassured me that he would be available if I changed my mind.

Five months later, my weight was still going up. The hot flashes and night sweats came back. And then I had the one set of symptoms I could not live with: vaginal dryness, friction, and atrophy. No amount of lubricant or foreplay could make the first sixty seconds of intimacy with the love of my life any less painful.

Suddenly, I was afraid to have sex.

It was no longer that I didn't want to, as with the loss of libido. I desperately wanted to. I wanted the closeness, the release, and the connection to my beloved. I wanted the orgasms. I wanted the fun, laughter, playfulness, and freedom of a healthy sex life. The irony was that twenty-one months after surgery I was still running from pain.

I called Dr. Bloch to see if I could start BHRT again.

Time to Rise

Physically, I was fine six weeks after my hysterectomy. I treated my surgery like I had six weeks off. I fell back into my life. I traveled on weekends, worked a normal schedule, biked, went to the gym, attended Toastmasters meetings, and socialized with family and friends.

But I was exhausted. I had jumped back into my life at full speed and intensity. It was too much too soon. In the past, pushing harder was all I knew. Now, I couldn't. Something had to give.

I began by giving up Toastmasters and evening activities. Next, I gave up morning activities, so I could sleep in. Giving up my job or taking more time off was not an option. Some women might have given up exercise. For me, giving up biking would have been like a death sentence. Cycling is my passion. It makes life worth living. To take that away from me, I'd have to be in therapy for years!

Months after my surgery, most people thought I was living a normal life and fully functioning. But to my inner circle, and especially to Jim, I wasn't myself. I was no longer calm and peaceful, and I certainly did not exude joy. Externally, I was functioning, but many times it felt like I was going through the motions on autopilot. Internally, I felt out of balance. My emotions continued their roller coaster ride, as did my energy.

During this time, it was Jim's job to keep his life in check. We are both strong, independent people. That said, we are better together, as we support, encourage, and inspire each other to be the best versions of ourselves. When we both feel good, life is amazing. When one of us is down, life is still beautiful, and, the other learns to pick up the slack. By down, I mean tired, injured, stressed, or even depressed. We both experience times where we are down. Fortunately, these are short lived, and we bounce back quickly. We also have learned that we can't both be down at the same time. That's our deal. And at this time, I wasn't ready to be up yet.

One week, I kept sinking deeper and deeper into my pity party and depression. The deeper I sank, the more Jim pulled away. In an emotional tirade, I lashed out at him verbally, accusing him of not being there to support me. I complained that when I needed him most, *he had disappeared.*

What ensued was a not-so-pretty "conversation" in which a lot of angry words were exchanged. One or both of us may have even said words we regretted. And one of us may have wrecked his car that day after storming out of the house and driving while upset. Hey, marriage ain't always pretty. But ours is honest, raw, and unashamed. Thankfully, we live by the agreement to talk things out and make it better. And we did.

Little did I know, Jim was doing everything possible to keep his life together. He felt alone, like he was going through life as a single person. *I had disappeared.* At this point, I had been down and out for over a year and a half. Jim had been carrying more than his weight in our marriage for that duration. It was time for me to rise.

There was a time to mourn, a time to cry, and a time to scream. There was a time to yell, a time to kick, and a time to release. And a time to rise. This was, indeed, the time for me to rise, to reclaim my joy and step back into my life boldly. It was time to make a comeback. It was time to come back strong.

The days immediately after that argument were probably the most difficult few days of our marriage. But it was a turning point for me. I had to take a hard look at my life and myself and decide whether I wanted to find a solution or wallow in my problems; to live life as a peaceful and joyful warrior or succumb to be a victim and alone.

I chose to rise. I chose to come back strong. I had mourned long enough. It was time to move on. After that wakeup call, I went to work on my mindset and habits. I became more conscious of my thoughts, words, and feelings. I guarded what I allowed into my mind regarding television, books, the news, social media, and relationships. Any area of toxicity got purged.

I combined everything I knew from traditional and nontraditional healing practices and I explored new paths and lifestyle changes to reduce stress and improve my life's balance and overall wellness. I worked to bring more peace and calmness to my life through meditation. I defined my definite major purpose. I uncovered passions and spent more time focusing on the positive. As I focused on happiness, balance and joy showed up.

And there was hope.

It took me close to two years to get where I am today, but now I mostly feel peaceful, balanced, energized, and free on a daily basis. I made a strong come back, and you can too.

CHAPTER 2

Preparing for Surgery and Initial Recovery

IN TALKING WITH WOMEN experiencing surgical menopause, I hear two common concerns: Some women wish they had been more prepared for surgery while other women were so afraid of the surgery that they did not educate themselves on what comes after: sudden surgical menopause. I didn't.

The most important part of preparing for surgery and your initial recovery is you. You are a critical part of the team. Stay empowered by playing an active role in your medical plan. This will help to alleviate some of the fear and anxiety about your surgery and can even speed recovery.

Your Personal and Family History

Before surgery, you will be meeting with one or more doctors, gynecologists, oncologists, anesthesiologists, pharmacists, and the like. The one person who can connect them as a team is you.

Wouldn't it be nice if our entire medical history were all in one place? That's how it is for Jim at the U.S. Department of

Veterans Affairs (aka the VA or DVA) that he's been with since his West Point days. Despite moving from New York to Georgia to Germany to Chicago to Ohio and back to New York again, the VA and his personal medical history followed him during and after his military career.

In my experience, that is not the case for civilians. Over the years, I have had multiple primary care physicians, gynecologists, gastroenterologists, acupuncturists, dermatologists, and other specialists located all over the country. My medical history and what each doctor knows is only as good as my personal records and what I share.

This is where we must become our own best advocates. Our doctors need to see us as whole people with our complete histories. They need as much information as possible to guide us, especially if we work with Eastern practitioners, such as acupuncturists or naturopaths, who follow the philosophy that everything is connected—no detail is insignificant. This includes a list of any prescriptions or over-the-counter medications, as well as vitamins and herbal remedies we take on a regular basis. Our doctors and pharmacists can advise us on anything we should stop taking before surgery and when it's safe to resume.

Our family medical histories also provide important clues that help doctors assess risk, schedule tests and screenings, and prevent and diagnose illness and disease. When possible, we should share as much information about our biological parents, siblings, and grandparents as we can gather, including any disease or health problems they may have and the ages and causes of their deaths.

Educate Yourself

Educate yourself on all options and alternatives, especially when it comes to surgery, drugs, and lifestyle changes. This book can help. It will be to your benefit to understand the:

- Natural progression of menopause.
- Suddenness of surgical menopause.
- Symptoms of menopause.
- Options for hormone replacement therapy.
- Difference between synthetic hormone therapy and BHRT.

In addition, understanding the many aspects of wellness and how surgical menopause can interrupt our sense of balance can help to keep things in perspective. These topics are covered in Chapter 3, "Wellness and the Challenges of Menopause." Having this basic understanding will help you communicate with your medical care team and make the best decisions concerning your health, surgery, and recovery.

Ask Questions

Remember, there are no stupid questions. Ask and keep asking. Some women don't know what questions to ask their doctors. Visit the Appendix for a list of suggestions. Take a written copy with you, so you don't forget any. The biggest question for me was how long would it take to recover. The answer: As long as it takes.

Second Opinion

It is perfectly acceptable to get a second opinion. When we seek guidance from another doctor, we are looking to confirm a diagnosis and/or find possible different treatment options. If our condition is not life threatening, then we have time to pursue less-invasive alternatives. With a cancer diagnosis, however, a hysterectomy can be lifesaving. Second opinions should be done quickly so an educated decision can be made and treatment can begin as soon as possible.

Take Notes and/or Bring a Friend

I admit I am not always the most objective patient. Hormones, diagnosis, and the prospect of surgery can cause me to be emotional and lose my perspective. Other women report going numb, tuning out large parts of conversations with doctors. When we are either emotional or numb, retaining critical information can be a challenge. I have found that when I invite a friend along, my friend provides an objective point of view, along with the opportunity to take notes.

Serenity Through Acceptance

Before surgery, I made three major decisions. I:
- Agreed to undergo surgery to have an ovary and fallopian tube removed.
- Trusted my doctor and husband to make the decisions that were in my best interest while I was unconscious.
- Promised to accept whatever outcome I woke up to.

Serenity is the state of being calm, peaceful, and untroubled. With serenity comes freedom. There are things that I cannot change: I no longer have a uterus or ovaries. We can't stuff them back in or do a transplant. I accept that. The uterus I wasn't using. The ovaries . . . well, that's another story, as they are headquarters for producing most hormones that keep a woman in balance.

There are things that I can change: my attitude, my feelings, my thoughts, my words, my habits, and my perspective. It takes courage and hard work, but I can change these things.

Learning to see and knowing the difference between what we cannot change and what we can is where the brilliance of the advice comes in. It is freedom. It is, indeed, serenity.

Every single one of us has adversity and challenges in life. So, the question for each of us becomes not whether we will have struggles, but how we are going to respond to them. As humans, one of our greatest skills is the ability to adapt and transform.

While there was serenity in accepting what I had no control over, I wanted to do everything within my power to go into surgery and initial recovery in the healthiest state possible. This included fortifying my body, choosing the right perspective, managing my expectations, reducing stress, and having a strong support network in place.

Fortify the Body

Some women will enjoy their favorite foods of pizza, ice cream, or a burger and fries before surgery. Because I am digestively challenged, I typically choose foods that are nutritionally dense and easy to digest. This was especially true before and after surgery. I drank lots of liquids to stay hydrated and prevent constipation, a common complaint after hysterectomy. I ate smaller, lighter, plant-based meals.

I was able to be active right up until the day of my surgery, but most exercise was off limits for six weeks afterward, so my body could focus all its attention on healing. My doctor told me I could walk as much as possible following surgery to help avoid blood clots and stiffness while promoting healing.

We all face surgery from different levels of health and fitness. If we've never run a day in our lives, we probably won't be running a marathon anytime soon. But we can begin today by making one positive change to our health. We can fortify our bodies to the best of our abilities.

Choose the Right Perspective

I believe perspective plays a huge role in how we enter menopause, regardless of whether it is natural or surgically induced,
as well as in how quickly we heal.

Think back to when you first got your period. What was
your perspective? Did you view it as an honor as you stepped
into womanhood, like my friend Susan? Or were you more like
my friend Stephanie, who viewed it as terribly embarrassing—
always having accidents and not being able to go in the water
at the beach for fear of bleeding through? For me, I understood
that getting my period made me a woman and enabled me to
have children. With my young naïve mind, I thought that the
day I got my period I would become pregnant. Silly? Or the
power of a child's brain who takes things literally?

What is your perspective of menopause? Is it a time of distress and discomfort? A signal of aging? Do you fear the best
years are behind you? Are you focused completely on your
symptoms? Or do you see this transition as a rite of passage
and a time to discover or rediscover your power, purpose, passion, and authenticity?

I love that the Chinese refer to menopause as the *second
spring*. They consider it a time to reflect on life and turn our
focus inward to nurture ourselves. That rings true for me, as
this season of my life already has had an ongoing theme of self-
love, self-care, and self-reflection.

Just like surgery may have benefits of alleviating pain or
risk of disease, menopause can be a wonderful transition with
positive side effects such as:

- No more periods, cramping, tampons, or pads.
- We can finally wear white pants again, any time of the
  month.
- We can enjoy sex without risk of pregnancy.

- We may have greater confidence and self-assuredness.
- We don't have to schedule our sex lives, athletics, or vacations around our periods.

After my surgery, it took time for my body to heal physically. It took even longer for my mind and emotional health to stabilize. There were times when I felt broken. I had to constantly remind myself that I was in a state of healing and change. Even though I felt broken, I told myself that I was whole, strong, and valuable.

Surgery and surgical menopause can be both frustrating and exhausting. The last thing we need to do is to beat ourselves up. And isn't that one of our greatest strengths as women? We think we should heal faster, we shouldn't cry for no reason and we should be able to do it all, even right after surgery. The only thing we need to do is cut ourselves some slack and remind ourselves that this too shall pass. That's a perspective I can embrace.

Managing Expectations

Along with a healthy perspective comes the ability to manage our expectations. This can include talking to our employers about options for time off. I was fortunate to receive short-term disability pay while I was out of work for six weeks. One woman I know took out a small loan to replace her paycheck, so she could take time off to fully heal.

Our expectations regarding the time it takes to feel good again require managing as well. There were times during my recovery from hysterectomy when I started to think that maybe I was imagining things. I wondered if, somehow, the plethora of physical symptoms and emotional fluctuations I felt were all in my head. *Maybe, menopause doesn't really exist.* After all, I spoke with other women who went right back to work within days of their surgeries and who appeared to have escaped surgical menopause altogether. Meanwhile, it seemed to take for-ever for me to feel normal again.

As I contemplated where this thought came from, I started to examine my expectations. Fifteen years prior, I stayed with my parents when my mom had a hysterectomy. The first days after she came home from the hospital, she was in physical pain, but aside from that, she escaped the added symptoms of menopause. Perhaps age played a factor: My mom was fifty-four when she had her surgery; I was forty-three. She had most likely already entered perimenopause, where the decline in hormones manufactured by her ovaries had already taken place gradually, so there wasn't such a sudden drop and change in her energy levels and emotions.

Being a sports nutritionist and having studied wellness for almost a decade, I also know how much our world has changed. The nutrient and toxicity levels of the foods my mom grew up with are different than the ones I've been exposed to. My generation has also been surrounded by more technology and radiation than any other generation in history.

It could simply be that everybody, even women within the same family, is different. My mother was lucky enough not to be affected by premenstrual syndrome, whereas my PMS symptoms had always been quite severe. I had endometriosis, which was not diagnosed until surgery. Add the complication of IBS with the endometriosis and it's no wonder I had a tougher time than my mom.

For those of us prone to anxiety, we worry and even have tendencies toward negativity and cynicism. In my experience, worry never resulted in anything good. In fact, it elevated my stress levels, made things worse, and slowed healing. I eventu-ally changed my expectation to one of positive optimism, and things began to get better. What I focused on grew. As I fo-cused on the good things in my life with gratitude, I found more in life to appreciate.

Another area of expectation that requires managing is post-surgery intercourse. I remember sitting in the doctor's office at my six-week checkup, discussing reentry into the world of sex. Jim and the doctor joked a bit as they sang a line of Madonna's "Like a Virgin." To warn you and to be frank, that's not quite accurate.

My first time after surgery felt like my vagina had shortened, shrunk, and dried up. While there is controversy over whether the vagina shrinks due to surgery, the reality is that our vaginas are resilient. They can, after all, bounce back after childbirth. Or so they tell me. They can bounce back after a full hysterectomy as well.

I found that the more relaxed I was, the less pain I had. I made sure I always had lubricant on hand and I used it early on to give my body all the help it required. This became a fun time of exploration as together Jim and I learned what got my juices flowing. Literally. For some women, it is soft music, candlelight, or a sexy movie. Others may enjoy this season of healing as a time to cuddle, talk, and explore other means of mutual pleasure and intimacy.

While we are on the subject of sex, let's talk about the libido. Sex and intimacy are not only physical. They are emotional. This is where desire comes in, otherwise known as libido. I once heard that when a man and woman fight, the woman needs to resolve the issue before she has sex. A man needs to have sex before he can resolve the issue. I say sex has a similar effect as exercise: If you ask me how my day was before a workout, you'll get a very different response than you will if you wait to ask me after.

When it comes to menopausal women, we are all over the board on this one. Some women are grateful for the "forced" break from intercourse that surgery provides. Perhaps they didn't enjoy sex or found it painful. If it's painful, it is natural to develop a fear of sex, which was my initial reaction. Then, there are others—and you know who you are ladies—who cannot wait to have sex. In their strong desire, they may even rush the process before their bodies are ready. This can cause harm and increases the risk of bleeding, infection, or torn stitches. I highly suggest waiting for the green light from your doctor.

Early on, I complained about a low libido. My doctor and I experimented with the addition of bioidentical testosterone. I fully expected BHRT to fix this, however, I did not notice significant improvement. I've known other women who tried testosterone and it made all the difference in improving their sex lives.

I kept an open mind and I recognized that sex brings a level of intimacy, communication, and relaxation to my marriage. I enjoy this closeness with Jim. So, I changed my expectations about BHRT and my mind about my libido. I took responsibility for my thoughts and feelings about my physical and sexual relationship. I embraced spontaneity as a grateful participant. I found that this approach always has a beautiful result: Orgasms bring joy, relaxation, and deeper connection. They also make me forget about my symptoms. And the laundry, the dishes, and anything on my chore list. Heck, sometimes I even forget my name.

As I took a closer look at my attitude and how it was related to my symptoms, I realized that it wasn't that I'd lost my libido at all. I'd lost my passion. But not for Jim or sex. For life. For my job. In fact, I was pleasantly surprised to discover that my libido was, in fact, strong. I also accepted that in my situation, it wasn't fair to expect BHRT to fix this. It was up to me.

Finally, remember that during recovery, our partners are going through their own transition, having their own emotions, reactions, frustrations, and expectations. They may attempt to be extra sensitive, not knowing if we are ready to be intimate or how we are feeling. It helps to keep the lines of communication open, especially in the initial recovery stage after surgery.

Physical release is part of a healthy lifestyle and it can certainly be a stress reliever. Men have needs, some more than others. They may choose to "release" on their own. I have heard some women say this makes them feel insecure, while others shame their partners about it. In the spirit of managing my expectations, I decided not to take it personally and to look forward to the time when it was safe and I felt good enough to join in.

Reducing Stress

Before surgery, I didn't recognize that I was stressed. Since then, I've discovered that there are two scenarios for stress. In one case, we know we are stressed. We are under a deadline at work, there's not enough money at the end of our month, the furnace breaks, a loved one is ill, we move, buy a home, get married, divorced, and so forth. Any major life event will cause stress and we usually see it and feel it. And we know it is temporary. The situation passes, and our stress levels drop. Hopefully.

The second scenario is where I found myself: with a cumulative buildup of stress that started with the initial discovery of a mass and a cyst. I was already leading a full and productive life that my body had adapted to. Or so I thought. But add in the stress of multiple surgical procedures, financial stress from a smaller paycheck while on short-term disability, and stress on my body as an athlete. Then add in the stress of constantly looking for a solution, to feel better, to lose weight, and to restore balance emotionally. And then, on top of that, add in the pressure I put on myself to race back to the same life as I knew it to be before surgery, and I was on overload. I was exhausted. I had to learn to relax, rest, and manage my schedule better. I had to remember how to play.

Now, I monitor my days so that I don't burn the candle at both ends, rising early and staying up late. I examine my vacation schedule to make sure I build in longer breaks and geta-ways. In between vacations, I take more naps and bubble baths. I enjoy a massage as often as I can. My bike rides are not all workouts; some are joy rides and playtime with friends. Yoga, meditation, spending time in nature, and doing things I love are all healthy ways to relax and calm my anxious mind and heart. These are some of the practices that help to reduce stress in my life. By the same token, I also had to learn to get off my own back. To allow grace and as much time to heal as I needed. The world won't end if I don't do the dishes tonight, finish the laundry, or take out the trash. That's what tomorrow is for.

A Strong Support Network

Having a strong support network will help you through sur-gery and initial recovery until you are back on your feet.

We know that relationships are important. After all, we are women. Our feminine nature is to connect and relate to peo-ple. There are studies about the advantages of strong, healthy relationships, and these benefits include living longer, being better able to deal with stress, improved physical health, feel-ing a richer better quality of life, lower rates of depression, better immunity, and improved blood pressure; things we can all benefit from as we navigate through surgery and surgical menopause.

You don't have to go through this alone. You may or may not have close family and friends. You may or may not be mar-ried or have a partner. Ask your doctors, employers, and health insurance company what resources are available to you for support. If you are on Facebook, there are wonderful groups composed of women just like you and me from around the world that share their experiences and what they have learned. These groups offer a safe place to discuss our fears and symptoms and ask questions. Two such groups are "Hysterectomy & Menopause Support Group" and "Surg Meno." Ask to join. I did.

I know reaching out to people is not always easy. In the past, I was a private person, to the point where I didn't share much about my health challenges with my parents or sister before surgery. In hindsight, I might have done this differently. My sister would certainly have wanted to pray for me. My mom would have just wanted to be there, offering support and encouragement while preparing meals, doing laundry, and cleaning my toilets. Some days, that's just what a girl needs from her mum—particularly right after surgery when your body is using all your energy for healing its tissues.

One way to receive support is to ask for help. My friend Holly knew a woman who had a hysterectomy and felt very alone. This woman needed assistance but did not know how to go about asking for help. Holly suggested she utilize social media. If she wanted a turkey sandwich she could post it on Facebook or tweet it on Twitter and have multiple offers within the hour. I love this idea. You could also ask for recommendations for people's favorite movie or book and invite some local friends over to watch with you or start a reading, writing, or coloring group.

Not everyone will know how to help us. This is where we need to communicate clearly by inviting friends, family, coworkers, and even neighbors into our lives. Let them bring a meal, do the dishes or a load of laundry, vacuum the floors, clean the kitchen, or pick up a few groceries. They can loan us movies or books, or drive us to the doctor or pharmacy. If we have children, they may help with childcare or transportation to afterschool events and play dates.

Or, they can come for a visit. Some days you'll want to talk, some days you'll want just to sit. Ask for what you need and accept what they can give. Release them if they can't. They will be there for you another time. Remember in the early stages of your recovery to let them know your energy limits so they can plan their time with you accordingly.

In the first weeks after my surgery, my friend Lucy brought me two puzzles while my friend Susan delivered a coloring book and colored pencils. I was amazed how fast time went by as I got lost in puzzle building and coloring. Both provided a healthy distraction from television, social media, and technology in general. They allowed my mind to relax, which resulted in calmness and clarity. Eventually, I was ready to have lunch with friends either at home or close by. When I walked, I invited friends to join me.

Know that your friends are not therapists or counselors and sometimes we require more of a listening ear than they can give. I found talking to a counselor played a large role in reducing my stress levels after surgery. I wish I had done it in the weeks prior to surgery as well.

An important part of the support network for some of us is our partner and/or our children. They get stressed too. During my recovery, Jim would act strangely or not quite like himself. I sensed it, and at times took it personally, until I realized not everything was about me. Laughter and lightheartedness were a great way to ease tension that surfaced.

Our men cannot read our minds. By nature, they have nothing in their lives to compare to hysterectomy or surgical menopause. As we go through surgery and experience the suddenness of symptoms after, we need to use our words to communicate our needs, desires, and fears. It may be as simple as asking for a hug or reassurance that they are with us through sickness, health, and menopause.

Clear communication is crucial with children as well. Include them in discussions about surgery and recovery. If they are old enough, they may be ready to take on more responsibility around the house. Children crave routine and familiarity and this is a time of change for your family. Try to keep their schedule consistent. Again, ask for help from family and friends. Let their teachers know what is going on so they can provide extra support. Above all, know that kids covet our time. Give them as much as you can, even if it is naptime.

Final Tips

As you prepare for surgery and your initial recovery, you might:

- Prepare and store meals (or collect them from family and friends).
- Make a list of local restaurants that deliver.
- Hire a house cleaner for the first few weeks after surgery.
- Schedule a driver to take you home after surgery.
- Plan childcare support while you are in the hospital and the initial weeks of recovery.
- Pick up extra books from the local library or order them for your Kindle.
- Sign up for Netflix.
- Go to the bank. Sign up for online banking and auto pay for recurring bills.
- Fill any prescriptions. Ask your pharmacy if they have a delivery service.
- Consider your home's layout. Can you avoid stairs or move things for easier access?
- Stop smoking. Smoking can cause complications with surgery and anesthesia. Talk to your doctor and consider stopping at least two weeks before surgery.
- Lose weight if necessary. Excess fat can cause complications with surgery and anesthesia and slow the healing process. Talk to your doctor or a nutritionist about the best way to go about losing weight before surgery.
- If you have other conditions, discuss them with your medical team to make sure they are well controlled. This includes diabetes, high blood pressure, anxiety,

and depression. The better managed they are before surgery, the less impact they will have after.

- Plan to take time off. Discuss all options with your employer as well as your family.

CHAPTER 3

Wellness and the Challenges of Menopause

AFTER SURGERY, I KNEW my body required time to heal. As the weeks passed by and I struggled to regain balance emotionally, I realized I wanted more than my physical health restored. Yes, I wanted to be free of pain and illness. I also wanted to be healthy on a mental, emotional, and social level. The goal was wellness. The obstacle was surgical menopause.

What Is Wellness?

Wellness is more than a state of health where you are free of illness. It is a state of well-being that is the result of deliberate effort. Wellness has its roots in alternative medicine and at its core it identifies the whole person as a collaboration of mind, body, and spirit.

I see wellness as a balancing act, much like riding a bicycle.

A bicycle is made up of two wheels composed of a tire, inner tube, and the wheel itself. The wheel is composed of an inner hub and outer rim, which are connected by a series of spokes. Bicycle spokes work together to support and evenly distribute the weight of the rider. On its own, a single spoke is easily bent. Put together with its fellow spokes and it supports a great deal of weight without bending. When one spoke does bend or break, all the other spokes take on more of the load. The extra pressure makes every other spoke more vulnerable to failure. In addition, damaged spokes can cause punctures to the wheel or get caught in your frame, causing you to fall. Every single spoke matters.

In life, just like on a bike, I've learned that it's important to keep my spokes in good working condition, so I can stay balanced and continue moving forward toward a life of wellness. The spokes in my wellness wheel include nutrition, exercise, faith/spirituality, relationships, finances, self-care/self-love, career, nature, prayer and meditation, rest, passions, purpose, play, and more. Together, they support my healthy lifestyle. When one of these areas or spokes is not working, all other areas are vulnerable.

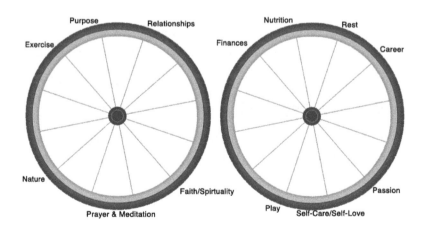

Before surgery, the spokes in my wheels to wellness were in pretty good condition. I was moving forward toward my goals and dreams with a sense of peace. Sure, at times one spoke or area would need a little extra attention. But in general, my ride of life was smooth.

When a woman begins to experience natural menopause, it may feel as if one spoke is bent or broken. She can focus on repairing it individually. When I experienced sudden surgical menopause, it felt like all my spokes were broken. Every single area of my life needed my attention. As I put each area of my life under a microscope, I dove into a world of self-discovery and awareness. I also began seeking solutions to regain my balance, so I could incorporate joy and peace.

I worked hard to minimize my symptoms and improve the quality of my health on all levels—physical, emotional, spiritual. I benefited greatly from the merging of both Western and Eastern practices and complemented both with other, self-designed lifestyle changes. I learned how intertwined my thoughts, words, and feelings were and I found tools to change them for the better. Wellness indeed took deliberate effort. This reclaiming of balance in my life did not happen overnight and to this day continues to be an ongoing balancing act.

So, if wellness is the goal and surgical menopause is the obstacle that breaks a spoke or two, or more, causing us to lose our balance and fall, then how do we fix these spokes, come back strong, and achieve balanced wellness after surgical menopause? It helped me first to understand the natural progression of menopause, the suddenness of surgical menopause, the symptoms that can come with both, the options for HRT, and the difference between synthetic and bioidentical hormones. Once I had this base understanding, I could then find tools through complementary medicine and lifestyle changes to manage my symptoms. When I went to work on my thoughts, words, and feelings, I gained even more strength of mind and balance of emotions.

The Natural Progression of Menopause

I speak with women in their forties or younger who complain about fatigue and suspect they might be fighting a cold. Others describe experiencing migraines or bitchiness at certain times of the month. Some have instances of vaginal dryness. What these women have in common is that they don't always put together that their symptoms are hormonal. They are in a state of premenopause or perimenopause.

What's the difference in these life stages? Premenopause arrives first. We may not even notice any changes in our bodies, minds, or moods, but our levels of estrogen and progesterone are beginning to drop. Perimenopause is next. Estrogen levels continue to drop and symptoms begin to arrive for the "party." Our period becomes irregular. Night sweats and hot flashes begin.

Menopause officially arrives when the ovaries stop releasing eggs.

Medically speaking, we have reached postmenopause when we have been without a menstrual period for over a year. We remain postmenopausal until the end of life, even if symptoms continue for months or even years.

My menstrual period ended at age thirty-eight, five years prior to the removal of my uterus. Due to heavy bleeding, I had an endometrial ablation, a procedure where the uterine lining is thinned causing the monthly menstrual period to stop completely, or at least for a while. By definition, I was *postmenopausal* since I hadn't had a period in over a year. However, since I still had my ovaries at that time, I felt the normal fluctuations of my hormone cycle.

The Suddenness of Surgical Menopause

When I used to hear the word *menopause*, I thought of hot flashes and older women. When I heard the words *surgical menopause*, I thought of hot flashes that start at an earlier age than normal. This was a very simplified version of what goes on with surgical menopause. These images were the only version of what might happen to me that I was aware of with my limited knowledge and perspective prior to my hysterectomy and oophorectomy.

Keep in mind that a hysterectomy itself does not include the removal of ovaries, and therefore will not send a woman into surgical menopause. An oophorectomy removes the ovaries and causes sudden surgical menopause.

The main difference between surgical menopause and natural menopause is the timeframe and intensity of the symptoms related to the transition. During natural menopause, symptoms appear gradually and are sometimes so subtle that we barely notice the changes; and when we do, we can tackle one or two symptoms at a time as they pop up.

My friend Theresa has been undergoing the process of natural menopause for the past couple of years. Her symptoms are not always consistent from month to month. Theresa recognizes that the severity of her menopausal symptoms is dependent on how well she's taking care of herself. Her stress levels, her workload, her sleep patterns, and her yoga practice, even her relationship with her son, all factor in.

By contrast, sudden menopause begins the moment the ovaries are surgically removed (oophorectomy) or are damaged by disease, radiation, chemotherapy, or other medications. This damage to or removal of the ovaries causes a sudden drop in estrogen and a deficit that will not be replenished due to missing ovaries and causes an immediate plunge into menopause.

If your ovaries were removed after menopause, you will not be in surgical menopause or feel any hormonal difference. If your ovaries were removed before menopause, then symptoms can show up abruptly, sometimes as soon as you wake up from surgery.

That is what happened to me. Although I was already post-menopausal by definition, once my ovaries were removed, a flood of symptoms appeared. I got hit all at once while I was recovering from major surgery. I had no time to adjust to the difference in my hormone levels and I suddenly felt off balance in my body and life.

While I felt quite out of sorts on many levels, I had decided not to have children many years before my hysterectomy. This is not the case for all women. I've heard from many women who felt a great loss when their reproductive organs were removed. There was a finality that caused intense feelings of emptiness and sorrow. They were questioning their decisions to have or not have children or to have more children.

I did find myself examining my past. I began looking to the future and I contemplated what I wanted to do with the rest of my life. It required patience as I dealt with these changes.

Leading Symptoms of (Surgical) Menopause

Suzanne Somers, aka Chrissy Snow from the sitcom *Three's Company* (1977–1984), has had success as an actress, author, singer, businesswoman, and health spokesperson. As an author, Somers offers great insights and reports from her interviews with many complementary and alternative doctors, in addition to her own experience with menopause. Somers gave me an education and a sense of humor as she wrote that menopausal "symptoms are like the Seven Dwarfs: itchy, bitchy, sleepy, sweaty, bloated, forgetful, and all-dried-up."[1]

Whether you go through natural or surgical menopause, you may get one of these, all these or none of these. Recovery is unique for each woman.

Itchy

As estrogen drops and hormone ratios change, a woman's body loses its ability to retain moisture. Skin, scalp, eyes, and vaginas are all areas where we can experience dryness. With dryness comes the itch. It is uncomfortable and equally embarrassing to be in a constant state of scratching.

Bitchy

In case you skipped the section where I describe how I yelled and cursed at the nurse in the hospital, that's what bitchiness looks like. Bitchy showed up at any time, without notice. It's like I was my very own version of Jekyll and Hyde, someone with two distinct and conflicting sides to my nature, fighting for center stage. I was not used to expressing anger, so this came as a bit of a shock to everyone around me, especially myself.

Sleepy

In the first weeks after my surgery, I was excessively sleepy. I thought that after six weeks, my energy would come back to normal. It took longer. And it took some troubleshooting. I had crashing fatigue where, out of nowhere, during my day I would "crash" and suddenly become extremely exhausted and fatigued both physically and emotionally.

Then, I developed a troubling case of insomnia. I couldn't fall asleep and on the rare occasion when I did fall asleep, I woke up every hour or two, never falling into the deep sleep that my body and mind craved. This deep sleep or non-REM sleep is where the body repairs and regrows tissue, builds bone and muscle, and strengthens the immune system. No wonder I was exhausted.

Now, when I don't sleep, I'm a mess; with surgical meno-pause, I was a hot mess. I became cranky, irritable, and suscep-tible to tears, outbursts, and illness. You've been warned.

Desperate for sleep, I decided to take advantage of a pre-scription for Ambien temporarily. Some women are reluctant to use pharmaceuticals or drugs of any kinds. It's a very per-sonal choice. From experience, I know that they can help dur-ing challenging times. I stayed open to solutions that got me through the toughest spots of surgical menopause. I made an educated decision and then I went to work on lifestyle changes that helped to alleviate my symptoms and rebalance my health. I eliminated coffee from my life (first after 12 PM, then after 10 AM, and finally, altogether). I turned off technology in the final hours before bedtime. I read to wind down, took soothing bubble baths, and learned relaxation techniques such as medi-tation. Eventually, through lifestyle changes and with the guid-ance of my medical team, I no longer required prescription drugs for sleep.

Sweaty

Hot flashes leave us dressing in layers, running the air condi-tioner on high, and wearing sleeveless shirts and flip-flops. During the winter. Night flashes have us kicking off the covers, pulling them back on, turning down the thermostat, then back up, opening the windows, closing them, freezing our partners out, then overheating them, and possibly driving them crazy in the process.

Fortunately, the small dose of BHRT that resolved my vag-inal dryness and atrophy also eliminated my hot flashes and night sweats. Some women who choose not to use hormones—whether bioidentical or other—report that acupuncture, nutri-tion, and other natural means can provide relief. Each body is different, and solutions are found through trial and error along with a healthy dose of patience and time.

For the period when I was not on BHRT, I found that a cooling pillow provided relief at night. Pillows, in general, can make a difference; some are designed to hold heat more than others. That goes for mattresses as well. Meditation helped with the hot flashes.

Bloated, Which Includes Weight Gain

As we age and estrogen levels drop, either naturally or induced, our body redistributes fat from our hips, fanny, and thighs to the abdomen. This belly fat results in the bloated-looking muffin top. Menopause is also a time when we gain weight, or at the very least, struggle to maintain the healthy weight we enjoyed in our younger years. It's too bad our hot flashes don't burn off calories and a little fat in the process.

As an elite athlete, I work hard to dial in my power-to-weight ratio that makes me effective as a cyclist. I am proud as a bodybuilder to be able to reduce my body fat. However, in the time leading up to my surgery and the months after, I gained an average of one pound per month for a total of twenty-five pounds. I spoke to other women who gained forty pounds in the year after their surgery. Our well-meaning doctors don't always know how to help us with this issue. Many of them will admit they only had a semester's worth of nutrition education. Nutrition is a critical piece to weight loss for women at any age and especially during menopause, as is stress reduction.

I found that people, including doctors, were unsympathetic to my complaints of weight gain. Friends would tell me I looked great, disregarding the fact that I didn't feel great in my body. Doctors would ask about my body mass index (BMI) and when I'd say it was high, they'd say, "No, it isn't." The reality was that while my BMI may have been acceptable, as an athlete my body fat percentage was high. This meant I was at a level where I didn't feel my best. Not to mention, gaining a pound per month over almost two years is not a pattern I wanted to continue or recommend.

As a wellness coach and sports nutritionist, I know what is required to lose weight. I understand the exercise component and know that for a woman weight loss is 60 percent nutrition and 40 percent exercise. After menopause, it probably jumps to 70 percent nutrition, 30 percent exercise. After surgical menopause, I'd bet it's closer to 80 percent nutrition, 20 percent exercise. So, while weight loss can be harder as we age or go through surgical menopause, it is not impossible.

My weight and body fat percentage did eventually come down. It was harder than in the past and slower, but not impossible. I recommitted to a nutrition plan, saving sugary treats for a special occasion, not an everyday response to overactive emotions. I changed my mind and my language. My words and thoughts had begun working against me. I blamed my weight gain on surgery and hormones and a now-slow metabolism. I said and thought things like, "I'm stuck," "I've plateaued," "My metabolism sucks," and "I can't lose weight." Then, I learned to keep my thoughts and words positive and affirming.

To this day, I work hard to speak positively about my body and myself. And I acknowledge myself for slow and steady progress in the direction I want.

Forgetful

I've heard women talk about senior moments as they age. I assume this might be the forgetfulness of menopause. For me, it was more like brain fog. As a writer, this was frustrating, as I felt my creativity was stifled. It was like I was never fully awake. I had trouble concentrating. Unfortunately, some of the traditional solutions I tried made the situation worse. For example, Ambien to help me sleep made it difficult to wake up in the morning, and consequently, I felt sluggish all day. I have learned to play detective, researching all medications and supplements, and even exploring nutritional deficiencies, as each of these can make brain fog worse. For example, I have taken antihistamines that exacerbated both my energy levels and fogginess. If I can reduce the need for them through diet, supplementation, and meditation, I can improve my clarity and focus. When I can find alternative solutions, it makes the symptoms of menopause seem less intense.

All Dried Up

Vaginal dryness can be an issue for women at any time, not just during surgical menopause. Increased foreplay can help increase blood flow to the vagina, assisting with dryness and libido. Other remedies can include lubricants, hormone replacement therapy, foods with phytoestrogens, and drumroll please . . . more sex!

No, I'm not kidding. When we get aroused, the blood circulation to our vaginal tissues increases, which stimulates the production of moisture. Abracadabra: no more dryness.

While I was certainly willing to try all remedies, the severity of this issue for me was the deal breaker that sent me back to BHRT. For other symptoms, I chose to look down other paths, in addition to being open to changing my perspective. It all boils down to this: What are you willing to live with? What would you like to live without?

Other Symptoms

Some additional menopause symptoms, which are no less aggravating, can include:
- Irregular periods.
- Hair loss or thinning.
- Dizziness or headaches and migraines.
- Incontinence.
- Increase in allergies.

- Changes in fingernails (weakening).
- Changes in body odor.
- Irregular heartbeat.
- Depression or anxiety.
- Breast pain.

Two of these symptoms that I want to address are depression and anxiety. Years before surgery, when I was going through a divorce, I needed a little bit of extra support. Lexapro got me through a rough few months. For me, it was not a long-term solution. I worked closely with my doctor and psychotherapist. They worked with the dosage and created a plan to wean me off medication when my emotions stabilized and after I had developed better coping skills.

Unfortunately, there can be a stigma or shame associated with taking antidepressant and anti-anxiety medication. I am neither pro-medication nor anti-medication. I believe there are times when they are essential and one of those times can be during surgical menopause when a woman's symptoms are at their worst.

I do believe that there are options that can lessen the severity or eliminate symptoms all together, such as hormone replacement therapy (HRT).

Hormone Replacement Therapy

Dean Bloch, M.D., is my primary guide and partner with HRT, as well as my OBGYN. Internists, family practitioners, and endocrinologists may also be in your toolbox to help balance your hormones. Dr. Bloch is patient and open to listening to my concerns while assisting me to feel my best. He sees me regularly, at times every three months, and we fine-tune my hormone levels based on my blood work as well as my symptoms and observations. HRT commonly includes estrogen, progesterone, and testosterone, or some combination of the three. HRT is used to replace or support the body's natural hormone levels. It is not just for surgical menopause, nor is it exclusive to women. My friend Natalie improved her libido in her thirties by taking testosterone, while my friend Tony began estrogen therapy after his diagnosis and treatment of prostate cancer.

Synthetic Hormone Therapy vs. Bioidentical Hormone Therapy

Synthetic hormones have been around for years in the form of Premarin, Provera, and even low-dose birth control pills. Synthetic means humanmade from chemical sources. I was surprised to learn that Premarin is produced from the urine of pregnant horses, or mares. Who knew? The goal is to create hormones that are similar, although not necessarily identical, to what your body naturally makes to alleviate symptoms. Many doctors prescribe synthetic hormones and many insurance companies cover the cost.

I was introduced to hormone, sexuality, and nutrition expert Camille Lawson, R.N., M.Ed., through a mutual friend. In a blog post entitled "Hormones: The Key to Vibrant Health and Sexuality for Women" she writes: "All bioidentical hormones originate from either soy or diosgenin (wild yam) plant sterols that are put through steps in a lab to become a hormone that is identical to the hormones manufactured by the body. Compounding pharmacies are key to correct formulation of your hormones, after a thorough hormone panel is done."[2]

Bioidentical hormones are humanmade and plant-based, however, they have the identical chemical structure as the hormones made by our ovaries. Bioidentical hormones are prescribed by a doctor and filled through a compounding pharmacy. The cost is most likely not covered by insurance. That said, my friend Tammy had an allergic reaction to synthetic HRT. With that diagnosis, she was able to switch to

BHRT and receive financial assistance from her health insurance company.

Bioidentical HRT was my choice. I also knew that I wanted a combination of some form of estrogen and progesterone for balance. I liked the idea that the hormone receptors in my body would recognize the yam extracts as familiar. BHRT ended up having a positive effect on my quality of life. Although at first, it didn't feel like it. I had to take responsibility for things in my life that required my attention. Counseling, mindset, discovering my purpose and passion, and allowing myself to do more of what I loved all played a significant part in my healing and recovery.

Even within wellness circles, there is a lot of controversy over the use of both synthetic and bioidentical hormones. Taking hormone replacements must feel right for you, your belief system, and your knowledge of health and safety.

The bottom line is, if you require HRT or BHRT or Ambien or Lexapro, or something else to eliminate night sweats, insomnia, anxiety, or depression, talk to your doctors. Explore your options and make an educated decision for this point in time. Then, go to work on lifestyle changes that help to alleviate your symptoms naturally and rebalance your health so that, under the guidance of your medical team, you eventually may not require pharmaceuticals.

CHAPTER 4

Complementary Medicine

SURGICAL MENOPAUSE BROUGHT ME a plethora of symptoms. At first, I wanted BHRT to fix everything. Dr. Bloch responded to my complaints and we continuously raised my level of hormones, to no avail. That's when I was forced to be more creative. I also took responsibility for what areas and symptoms I could positively impact.

The following list of tools includes modalities that I turned to before, during, and after surgery and menopause. These alternative forms of medicine are nontraditional in the sense that they are treatment approaches and practices that are not generally taught in medical school or available in hospitals. They may or may not be covered by insurance. They are, however, rooted in ancient beliefs and healing practices. These complementary medicines view the mind and body as a connected system and can help you to achieve more balance in your life and overall wellness. As I used complementary medicine and made changes to my lifestyle and mindset, I found a smaller dose of BHRT worked wonders. Fortunately, my doctor was open to this solution as well.

Acupuncture

Acupuncture is a medical protocol for balancing energy in the body and has been known to prevent, diagnose, and treat disease, as well as to improve general health.

I discovered the benefits of acupuncture over five years before surgical menopause. From my earliest appointments, my local practitioner, Carolyn Rabiner, L.Ac., Dipl. C.H., spoke to me about balance. My lifestyle had a lot of yang (active/masculine) energy. Yin (receptive/feminine), not so much. I have a feeling I'm not alone. If you are a work hard/play hard personality, your energy constitution is most likely the same. I've heard other women say, "I'll sleep when I'm dead." We push and push, staying up late, getting up early. We don't rest. We work hard. We work harder. And when our schedule overflows, it is the yin activities, like yoga and meditation, that get dropped. Slowly, the accumulative effects of stress start to manifest in illness, anger, and frustration. We find ourselves burned out, overwhelmed, fatigued, and screaming at our kids, partners, loved ones, coworkers, employees, and friends. And then, a life event like surgical menopause pushes us beyond   our limits.

Before we get to this point, however, we have options. Things we can do to restore our balance. Balance was something that Dr. Rabiner guided me to seek. Yes, I could be an elite athlete, and I also needed to listen to my body and seek harmony through counterbalancing activities, such as yoga, quiet walks, meditation, and qigong. When I mentioned that my symptoms decreased when I spent time writing, her advice was to keep writing. After long absences from writing on my part, I would show up on her table, feeling desperate and overwhelmed, claiming that my body didn't know how to heal or rebalance itself. She would gently remind me that it did.

Acupuncture aims to treat and address problems at their root cause. According to Dr. Rabiner: "Among other benefits, acupuncture has a major effect on the dynamics of blood circulation, assists the body in the process of the elimination of toxins, helps to greatly reduce stress levels, has an anti-inflammatory effect, and helps to restore normal function to the hormonal system. This can help women recover more quickly from the problems associated with surgical menopause."

Acupuncture can assist women with natural or surgical menopause. It can help to:

- Lessen the side effects of surgery, anesthesia, and pain medications.
- Reduce pain.
- Decrease reliance on opioids prescribed after surgery.
- Reduce anxiety, depression, migraines, fatigue, and gynecologic disorders.
- Promote overall well-being.
- Treat the post-traumatic stress that can arise from surgery or during sudden surgical menopause.
- Control chemotherapy-induced nausea and vomiting.
- Reduce the frequency of symptoms that occur during menopause, such as hot flashes and night sweats.

Herbalism

According to the American Herbalists Guild, herbal medicine is both an art and a science, one that uses herbs not only to promote health but also to treat and prevent illness. This is not a new practice; it has a 5,000-year-old history. Furthermore, pharmaceuticals were originally derived from plants. Today, you'll find herbalists, acupuncturists, naturopaths, midwives and everyday people using herbs for wellness. It is common in traditional Chinese medicine (TCM), Ayurveda (the indigenous medical system of India and Nepal), and naturopathic medicine. Herbs are safest when used by a trained herbalist.

My first recollection of herbal medicine was with St. John's wort. While I didn't take it myself, I heard a coworker describe taking it for its antidepressant qualities. It also has potent anti-inflammatory properties, which is key to healing after surgery.

Years later, I was introduced to a nutritional cleansing program that quickly became a staple in my daily diet. One supplement I take daily for its combination of adaptogens (plants that can help your body adapt to physical, chemical, and environmental stress, and balance normal body functions), antioxidants, and nutrients. I have been known to chase away a case of the moody blues with an extra shot of Ionix® Supreme. This daily elixir has ingredients such as rhodiola rosea, ashwagandha, eleuthero, schisandra, maca, and more.

Andrew Weil, M.D., is an internationally recognized expert in integrative medicine, a field that approaches healing the body, mind, and spirit. According to his website, www.drweil.com:

- Rhodiola can help increase energy, lower cortisol, fight depression, improve brain function (focus and memory), and burn belly fat.
- Ashwagandha can relieve anxiety, depression, and stress, increase stamina, alertness, and endurance, and stabilize blood sugar.
- Eleuthero or "Siberian ginseng" has been found to reduce lethargy, fatigue, and low stamina.
- Schisandra is used with cases of spontaneous sweating and to promote strength and stamina.
- Maca root is used to treat depression and low libido.
- Arnica can be used to treat physical trauma.
- Black cohosh is used for relief of hot flashes
- Dong quai or "female ginseng" has been used for low vitality, fatigue, and inflammation.

Massage Therapy

Massage may not be your first thought for managing your menopausal symptoms, but it has a multitude of benefits, including the release of feel-good endorphins, which help in alleviating headaches, reducing stress, regulating the body's fluid balance, and balancing hormone levels.

According to Michelle Renar, LMT, CEIM, massage therapist and owner of Hudson Valley Body Works in Kingston, New York: "Menopause can be an extremely tumultuous time in a woman's life. This can be especially true for women who are going through premature, medically induced menopause. Massage therapy with a skilled practitioner in conjunction with therapeutic essential oils can be an enormous help with the transition. Safe touch has a power no pharmaceutical company can ever reproduce."

Counseling

Surgical menopause is a life-changing event, one that can cause the desire to heal past hurt, examine present frustrations, and reveal future dreams. This can cause feelings of anxiety, depression, or uncertainty. The right psychological counselor can provide tools to help process these strong emotions before and after surgery. Psychologists, marriage and family therapists, and social workers are all trained to do individual therapeutic counseling sessions. Also, most insurance plans cover the cost if you find a counselor within your specific plan.

Six months after surgery, a therapist asked me how it felt when I knew I had survived the surgery. I remember screaming at him in frustration, "I haven't survived it." He gently reminded me that I had. I survived because I woke up after surgery. I was alive and mobile and highly functioning. What I required was to uncouple—to disconnect and release—the surgery from the symptoms in my mind, as well as my emotions.

Another counselor showed me how truly powerful words are. We can speak words that build up and empower, or we can speak words that tear down and destroy. This applies to ourselves and everyone around us. For years I told myself that I was not a good verbal communicator. I believed it, especially during surgical menopause when I tried to explain what I was going through. In one session, I mentioned this. I even apologized to my counselor for not being clear in my speech. Shari smiled and said, "My dear. You are a great verbal communicator. I understand exactly what you say."

And I believed her.

In one moment, speaking positive words changed a belief I had about myself. In his book *The Four Agreements*, don Miguel Ruiz talks about the power each of us has: "Each human is a magician and we can either put a spell on someone with our word or we can release someone from a spell."[3] I believe that is why Shari's words were so powerful over me. Her spoken words released me from lies I had told myself that simply were not true.

Chiropractic

Chiropractic care is not just for the back or neck. Proper alignment can help the entire body function better by helping to balance the nerves that help the body relax. When the body is relaxed, we experience better sleep, clearer thoughts and improved vitality, all beneficial outcomes when dealing with menopause, both surgical and natural. Chiropractic care can even lower elevated levels of cortisol and other inflammatory hormones, helping to further balance hormones and promote healing.

Chiropractic adjustments can be a safe, non-pharmaceutical alternative in treating menopause. There are areas of the lumbar spine and sacrum that directly affect the sympathetic and parasympathetic systems, which oversee hormonal regulation and can further assist during menopause. I have certainly experienced less hormonal headaches from chiropractic care, and other women have shared with me their benefits of less bloating, cravings, and cramping after their visits with their chiropractors.

How a Day at the Beach Provides Relief

On our first vacation together, Jim introduced me to the beach. Sure, I had grown up around boats, lakes, and canals. But as an adult, I hadn't gone to the beach to relax. At first, I wasn't sure I could do it. I usually seek adventure and love to play. But all it took was one day next to the ocean and I was hooked.

The summer after my surgery, my friend Susan and I snuck away for a day at the Jersey Shore. It provided relief from all that I had been feeling. A day by the tide left me relaxed and refreshed.

I've come to realize this doesn't just happen by the ocean. It happens in nature and near water in general. I decided to do some research to find out why. It is all about negative ions and their positive effect on our health. Here is the science behind how a day at the beach provides relief for our menopausal symptoms. If you don't love science, then skip the next paragraph. Better yet, head to the beach. For us science geeks, read on. And then, head to the beach.

Ions are invisibly charged molecules made up of an unequal number of electrons and protons. This gives a molecule a negative or positive charge. Ironically, positive ions can be harmful to our health, whereas negative ions are beneficial. Our environment is filled with those harmful positive ions in polluted cities, confined spaces, and technologically exposed environment. Negative ions are abundant in less developed areas and can improve our moods, immune systems, and sexual drives. They can provide relief from allergies and help us feel less drowsy and more alert and focused. I found that when I exposed myself to more negative ions through nature, my menopausal symptoms were less noticeable. That was reason enough for me to head outdoors.

In my quest to understand negative ions, I discovered another option: Himalayan salt lamps. These lamps, comprised of a large piece of pure, pink Himalayan salt with a lightbulb inside, can be placed in the home to help neutralize the positive ions created by electronic devices. While I can't get to the beach every day, I can benefit from the negative ions of a salt lamp in my home and office.

CHAPTER 5

Lifestyle Changes

MENOPAUSE, EVEN THE SURGICAL kind, is not a disease. A woman's body was created to go through this transition naturally, without interference. Things that can help lessen or alleviate symptoms include exercise—aerobic, weight-bearing, and flexibility—proper nutrition, rest, and consistent effort to reduce stress.

I was willing to shift my lifestyle and change some of my habits to help reduce and alleviate my different surgical menopause symptoms. Overall, these changes allowed me to feel more balanced in wellness.

Exercise Your Body

Exercise can have powerful benefits before, during, and after menopause, regardless of whether it is natural or surgically induced. My doctor cleared me to walk just days after surgery, but it was six weeks before I could do cardiovascular, strength, or flexibility training.

Fitness experts recommend exercising aerobically three to five times per week for twenty to sixty minutes. Add in weight-bearing exercise two times a week, focusing on strengthening all major body parts. Flexibility can be accomplished through active stretching or yoga. This may be the goal in wellness, but as we recover from surgery, we'll want to ease into it gradually.

Exercise has always helped me to relieve stress and release excess energy. Cycling was and continues to be a tool that helps me through the stress and hormonal fluctuations of menopause. Strength training allows me to maintain and build lean muscle, which helps to speed up my metabolism, which helps with weight management. I have found that when it comes to exercise, it is most important to find what you love and then to do it with consistency. You may need to explore a few things to discover what that is for you.

As I eased back into fitness, the first step was to start building healthy habits. There were days when all I had the energy for was a five-minute walk. So, I did that. And I did it every day, multiple times. I made it habitual. Every day or so, I added another minute in duration.

I know a woman who, when she was recovering from her hysterectomy, joined a fitness class for older adults. She was the youngest in the group, but she made some great friends, some of whom previously had experiences like hers: surgical menopause. She found the class to be just the right place to ease back into fitness. The instructor was even able to provide modifications to movements in consideration of her sensitive abdomen area.

When I was cleared to begin strength training, I had mixed emotions. I was both excited and scared. I had this image that my insides were going to fall out. Then I remembered I didn't have anything left to fall out. So, I went to the gym. I started small and used very light or even no weight. The first few weeks the most important thing was to show up for my workout and reestablish the habit in my schedule. I was patient with myself and gradually my strength and endurance came back, stronger than ever.

It is natural to feel intimidated when starting an exercise program even without the symptoms of menopause. I find working with a personal trainer to be extremely helpful. Many trainers will offer introductory specials to help you get started. Fortunate for me, I'm married to one.

Jim likes to joke that in all areas of life, I'm the boss. His only demand . . . er . . . *request* . . . is that he's the boss in the gym. And I gladly let him. In the gym, I trust his guidance.

Trust is the key factor in any relationship, but especially with your doctor and other healthcare providers and personal trainer. A good personal trainer can help you before surgery, and then again once your doctor gives you the green light to exercise. Your trainer can create a customized program that balances cardiovascular, strength training, and flexibility exercise. All three are important at this time in your life to build muscle and strength, burn body fat, and rev your metabolism.

Exercise also gave me a boost in confidence. Pole fitness helped me feel sexy again. Likewise, hula hoop, belly dance, and aerial silks workouts can do the same. There is something graceful, captivating, and attractive about these forms of exercise. There are times in life when we just don't feel sexy. But there's no reason we can't feel good in our bodies and about our sexuality after surgery and throughout the various stages of menopause. This is especially true if we struggle with weight gain.

Finally, flexibility training can help prevent injury, alleviate back pain, and assist with balance and range of motion. And it certainly helped to ease some of the stiffness I had post-surgical rest and recovery.

Nutrition

Every day our bodies require vital nutrients to function. Before and after surgery we can eat foods that are easy to digest and whose anti-inflammatory properties help our bodies heal. We can use nutrition to maintain or lose weight. Certain foods can minimize our menopausal symptoms, while others, such as caffeine, can exacerbate them.

Nutrition to Support Healing

An anti-inflammatory diet is well balanced and something anyone can benefit from, but especially someone preparing for or recovering from surgery. Inflammation is the body's way to heal after trauma. It brings increased blood supply and nutrients to the affected body part and helps to fight off infection. Its sole purpose is to repair. So, in the short-term, inflammation is good. Long-term inflammation is what we want to avoid, as it starts to damage healthy tissue.

There are two aspects to an anti-inflammatory diet.
1. Eat fruits, vegetables, whole grains, and fish
2. Avoid high-carb, low-fat foods

Some top healing foods that will reduce inflammation and speed post-surgical healing include green leafy vegetables, bok choy, celery, beets, broccoli, blueberries, pineapple, salmon, bone broth, walnuts, coconut oil, chia seeds, flax seeds, turmeric, and ginger.[4]

Foods that cause inflammation as they elevate insulin and glucose levels include flours, sugars, corn oil or peanut oil, pastries, cakes, and margarine.

You don't have to sacrifice flavor by eating more anti-inflammatory foods. To avoid excess sugar and salt, I experiment with flavor enhancers such as garlic, onion, ginger, turmeric, rosemary, cloves, nutmeg, and cayenne.

Nutrition to Maintain or Lose Weight

Weight gain is a common complaint from women in menopause. As a wellness coach, I know what to do to lose or maintain weight. Even so, I still gained weight with surgical menopause. Losing weight is not always easy, but it is possible, and it starts with nutrition.

Here are a few tips to assist you with managing your weight.

- *Drink more water.* Drink half your body weight in water daily. Add eight ounces for every twenty minutes of cardiovascular exercise or thirty minutes of strength training. Add additional water if you drink coffee or alcohol, if it is hot out, or if you sweat excessively.

- *Eat smaller meals more often.* Three hours after a meal, blood sugar levels begin to fall. At four hours, your body has digested what you previously ate. Hit the five-hour mark and your blood sugar plummets and you will likely grab whatever you can to refuel. To avoid this, plan to eat at least five meals a day, eating one meal every two to three hours. Finish your last meal three hours before bedtime.

- *Eat more protein.* There was a time when a typical breakfast for me was a bagel and coffee. I have since learned that every single moment, even when at rest, the body is breaking down and building up protein. And protein is the building block of muscle. At any point in time, our bodies are either building muscle or building toward fat.

- *Eat more vegetables.* Vegetables provide an assortment of nutrients. The more variety of colors, the wider variety of nutrients we get. I add spinach or broccoli to eggs, build a salad, or stir fry with the goal of having a rainbow of colors—topped with a lean protein.

- *Flavor with herbs and spices.* We train our taste buds to enjoy high-sodium, high-sugar, gluten-filled, and processed foods. We can just as easily train them to like healthy foods. Consider a "fast" from sauces, salt, and sugar. Instead, choose flavor from pepper, garlic, onion, and cumin. Add cilantro and dill to your salads. There is a whole world of herbs and spices that will tantalize your taste buds. You may even try foods plain—and realize you love their natural taste—especially as you reduce your sugar and salt intake.

- *Have a plan.* When I have a plan, I avoid emotional eating. At night, I plan and prepare my meals and snacks for the next day. A healthy afternoon snack helps me avoid the vending machine and other office goodies. If friends gather for happy hour, I plan to be the designated driver or opt out of drinking alcoholic beverages. If a friend asks to meet over a meal, I suggest an alternative that does not involve food: a walk or hike, or a new yoga class. Other options to suggest are hitting the batting cages or playing mini-golf.

- *Be prepared.* I cannot always predict where I will be at the time of my next meal, or if healthy options will even be a choice. I stay prepared by carrying the necessities: water, healthy snacks and even a meal on the go such as a high-quality protein shake or meal replacement bar.

Nutrition to Minimize Menopausal Symptoms

According to the weight-loss blog Eat This, Not That, there are several things we can eat and drink to help us age gracefully and minimize menopausal symptoms.[5]

- *Water.* Staying hydrated helps women to avoid dryness, itch, and bloat.
- *Flaxseeds.* Flaxseeds are beneficial during hormonal changes due to their estrogen-like compounds. Store them in the refrigerator and grind just before eating.
- *Almonds.* Almonds are a healthy fat and can counter the drying effect of low estrogen.
- *Eggs.* Eggs are a good source of vitamin D, iron, and B vitamins for energy as well as strong bones.
- *Green leafy vegetables and blueberries.* Both green leafy vegetables and blueberries are foods that fuel the brain. Think kale, swiss chard, collard greens, and lettuces.

Naturopath, chiropractor, and certified nutrition specialist Josh Axe also suggests foods such as broccoli, cabbage, kale, nuts, seeds, legumes/beans, avocado, wild-caught salmon, halibut, sardines, coconut milk, kombucha, and sauerkraut to help manage menopausal symptoms.[6]

In addition to the list above, nutritional cleansing and replenishment helped my body recover from all it had been through related to surgery: the tests, the X-rays, and the stress, both physical and mental. A side benefit was weight loss. While I wanted to cleanse the bad out, I also want to make sure I was bringing superior nutrients into my body: vitamins, minerals, essential amino acids (the nine that cannot be made by the body, but must come from food), and phytonutrients (chemical compounds from colored vegetables and fruits).

Foods that Exacerbate Menopausal Symptoms

According to the women's wellness blog 34MenopauseSymptoms, there are five main foods and drinks to avoid when struggling with menopause symptoms.[7]

- *Salty processed foods.* Extra salt will cause fluid retention, which leads to bloat. It can also increase blood pressure, leading to diseases that can complicate menopause symptoms.
- *Alcohol.* Alcohol can trigger headaches, anxiety, hot flashes, and night sweats, all common complaints during menopause.
- *Spicy foods.* Hot peppers and other spicy foods can trigger hot flashes and night sweats.
- *High saturated fat and sugar.* Foods like white bread, pie, cookies, muffins, and cake can cause blood sugar to spike as well as weight gain. My friend Lucy, who is a Catholic, gave up sugary sweets for the six weeks of Lent one year. After Easter, she snuck a treat from her child's Easter basket. She started getting headaches about the same time, and it took three times doing this before she connected the headaches to adding sweets back into her diet. What a great life lesson from the Easter basket, especially if one of your symptoms of menopause is migraine headaches.
- *Caffeine.* Coffee and soda can interrupt our natural energy and sleep patterns.

Fatigue is a common complaint of menopausal woman and caffeine is a common response. Therefore, what I'm about to tell you may cause alarm, fear, disbelief, and absolute rebellion, but if you are willing to try this simple solution, you may find yourself sleeping better, experiencing less anxiety, and getting over the roller coaster of energy highs and lows you live with. For good. I know I did.

The year after my surgery, I found myself having trouble sleeping, another common symptom of menopause. It may have been my wired mind, menopause, adrenals, stress, or any combination of things. Anyone who has trouble sleeping will tell you: It sucks. Yes, I'm the all-natural girl, but as I mentioned earlier, I did fill my prescription for Ambien back then, and alas, I did use it. Every last little pill.

What made the biggest, long-term difference was giving up my morning cup of "joe." This is a controversial subject. I wish I had a $1 for everyone who has said to me "I've already given up every other vice. I'm not giving up my coffee." Yes, they use the term *my*. They own it. It is their possession. Which borders on *obsession*.

I get it. I truly have exhibited all the behaviors of an addict when it comes to coffee. I was willing to give it up for my health and well-being, especially when fatigue was one of the predominant menopausal symptoms. Relief did not happen overnight. It got worse before it got better as my body slowly released this chemical from my cells. But I'm happy to say, it is no longer part of my daily routine, and I'm now falling asleep easier and staying asleep longer.

As I transitioned away from coffee, I found two natural drinks that brewed and tasted very much like my beloved coffee: Teeccino® and Dandy Blend. I also found I love herbal tea.

It took close to three weeks for me to feel the full effect of life without caffeine. But it had a drastic effect on my energy levels. Ironic, isn't it?

I believed that caffeine gave me an energy boost, but the reality was that it was contributing to my fatigue. With each cup of coffee, I was borrowing energy from the future. The problem was, I was never replenishing it with rest and sleep, which left me frazzled, overtaxed, overwhelmed, and anxious. Caffeine is a chemical stimulant, not a source of true energy. This "energy" is on loan from the adrenals and liver.

Check out some more of the negative effects caffeine has been associated with: irritability, mood swings, panic, and anxiety, anger, sleep disturbances (quality and duration), PMS, fatigue, depression, hormonal imbalance, headaches, gastrointestinal distress, increased stress, and reductions in iron and calcium absorption. It also increases the appetite for sweets and fatty foods, resulting in weight gain. It can even decrease levels of estradiol (the primary form of estrogen in our bodies) and testosterone, thereby throwing off the delicate balance of our hormones and affecting our libido, strength, power, and zest for life.

I struggled with many of these symptoms before giving up coffee. However, I found that as I removed caffeine and sugar from my diet, my cravings for them decreased. My energy improved, I experienced better digestion and sleep, fewer headaches and bloat, and weight loss. I noticed a difference in my ability to concentrate as well as my emotional response to include anger, irritability, mood swings, and depression. Not to mention, I saved a few bucks every week from not buying coffee, which always helps to reduce stress.

Rest

Surgery did one thing for sure: It took me down. I was forced to rest, which was a good thing. Good, but not always easy for a type A personality like me. I work hard, and I play hard. I've now learned to rest as well. In athletics, there is an intensity-to-recovery ratio. The more intense your workout, the more recovery is required. Think of surgery as an extreme workout for your body, mind, and emotions.

If I'm honest with myself, life before my hysterectomy was lived at 180 miles per hour. I have since learned that a balanced life requires—even demands—rest and recovery on a daily basis. I cannot wait for an annual vacation to take a break. I require timeouts on a quarterly, monthly, weekly, and daily basis.

This is where I take time to tune out the world and relax, play, and release the stress of everyday life. It is a time to rest, recover, reflect, and bring my life back into balance. I had to learn to make this a regular aspect of my healthy lifestyle, not a quick fix. When my body is tired and my spirit weary, the best thing I can do is rest.

Signs that would indicate you may not be recovering from surgery or that surgical menopause is taking a toll on you include:

- Difficulty waking up in the morning.
- Requiring more stimulants (caffeine, sugar) to keep going.
- Utilizing alcohol, sleeping pills, or other substances to wind down or fall asleep.
- Exhibiting a shorter fuse than normal, especially with loved ones.
- Lack of focus, creativity, or productivity.

To become more aware of what areas of life might need some extra attention, you can ask yourself the following questions.

- "Am I fueling my body with the proper nutrients?"
- "Am I sleeping enough? Do I require a nap?"
- "When was the last time I had a date night? Family day? Time with a friend?"
- "When was the last time I got lost in a good book or a movie?"
- "Can I give myself a creative outlet through writing, music, dance or art?"
- "Do I need to unplug from the computer, phone, or social media?"
- "Have I taken a day, weekend, or week off lately?"

- "Are my vacations becoming staycations, where I work so hard around the house that I have to go back to work to rest?"
- "Have I rejuvenated at the beach, by the lake or an ocean, in the mountains, or elsewhere in nature?"
- "When was the last time I laughed?"
- "Is my schedule too full? Where can I build in rest and recovery?"

If you find yourself less focused, creative, friendly, or productive, as I did, it may benefit you to slow down or take a break. As our intensity-to-recovery ratio improves, we are better able to come back stronger, more creative, productive, and refreshed, and with renewed energy and excitement. We have more passion for our career, relationships, and life in general. We'll find we are balanced through the transition of menopause.

Sleep

Sleep is a major part of rest and recovery, especially after surgery. It is also one of the most underrated yet critical aspects of our health and hormones.

After surgery and despite my case of insomnia, my body required more rest and sleep to heal and recover, and it took longer than I thought it should. However, I learned to listen and allow myself more grace for what was required: mornings without pressure, a chance to snuggle into the covers, burrow my head like an animal in its den, and allow healing and recovery to take place for a little longer.

Now, I'm not naturally a napper. In the past, when I hit afternoon fatigue or feel an energy crash, I would deny it. I'd stuff it back in. Carry on, warrior! But often this made situations worse. I noticed that the more caffeine I consumed, the harder I pushed, and the more wound up, anxious, and irritable I got.

I no longer ignore my body's signals to rest. I take a nap. I don't feel guilty. It usually only takes twenty minutes and I awaken feeling remarkably better and ready to conquer the world, or at least my small part of it. Ah, the restorative benefits of sleep. It is where the body does its best repair work.

In addition to napping, evening rituals benefit the quality and quantity of my sleep. I keep the final hour or two before bedtime sacred. I turn off all electronics, including television, computer, and phone. As the sun goes down outside, I begin to dim the lights inside. I take a bath, read, or meditate. Lavender essential oil helps me to relax, as does chamomile tea. I also use a melatonin sleep spray. Melatonin is a hormone we naturally produce that helps us sleep, providing feelings of relaxation. When the levels are correct, it allows us to naturally rest at night for twelve hours and wake up with ease.

Magnesium is a supplement that is critical for regulating melatonin and calcium is beneficial for undisturbed sleep. I take both. I have also been known to drink tart cherry juice to help me fall asleep. Why? Because tart cherries assist with serotonin production, which is necessary for the body's natural production of melatonin. Other foods that do this include bananas, oats, tomatoes, and pineapple.

An interesting fact I learned from John Gray, author of *Men Are from Mars, Women Are from Venus*, is that men relax in front of the television while women relax reading. It's how our brains are wired. Jim and I enjoy being next to each other, or at least in the same room. But I am grateful for the headphones he bought so he can continue to relax and unwind watching television. They mean I can be in the same room as him, reading in silence before bed.

One additional all-natural tool I use for relaxation and sleep is an acupressure mat. I've heard this referred to as a "bed of nails" and when I first laid my naked back down on this foam mat with hundreds of sharp, short, plastic needles, that's what it felt like. It seems counterproductive, but after the initial shock of the "needles" my body and mind relax, and I drift off.

Stress Reduction

Chronic stress that goes untreated can affect body, mind, and emotions. Mine also made my menopausal symptoms worse. To find balance and avoid burnout, I had to find ways to reduce stress.

A somewhat newly recognized complication of surgical menopause is adrenal fatigue. The adrenals are two endocrine glands that sit above the kidneys and produce hormones like adrenaline and cortisol. These hormones are so critical to our well-being that being depleted of them, as we become during long periods of continuous stress, can multiply our symptoms on top of surgical menopause.

Adrenal fatigue occurs when the accumulative effect of stress starts to manifest with illness, anger, frustration, and overwhelm. Suddenly, we find ourselves burned out and fatigued. We scream at our kids, partners, loved ones, coworkers, employees, and bosses. We damage relationships. I found myself experiencing all these symptoms in the months after surgery. The longer I experienced symptoms of surgical menopause without relief, the worse they seemed to get.

Our health is affected by the decisions we make daily. Stress is often not a result of one factor, but the cumulative effect of many factors. It helps me to look at what I can control now. In this moment, I may not be able to leave a stressful job, but I can decide not to eat the cookie someone has offered me or reach for caffeine to get me through my day.

I've also learned to say no more often, especially to things that don't align with my healthy goals, purpose, passion, and priorities. Some weeks I still cross off the morning and evening hours on my calendar and schedule those as sacred "me" time. I do my best to create good habits with food and exercise, and I now build in time to rest and recover, practice yoga, and meditate.

These are all part of my system of self-care that helps to reduce stress, alleviate symptoms, and bring me back into balance. As a woman I tend to put others first, to my own detriment. This leaves me compromising on my needs, especially when it comes to relaxation and self-care. After surgery and during surgical menopause it was important to make myself a priority. I learned what I required to relax, and I asked my family to adjust.

Yoga

Yoga is a major support in stress reduction for me. It helps me to calm my body, which in turn, quiets my mind. In the past few years, I have explored many different forms of yoga and I'm still learning. When I take care of myself and practice yoga even once or twice a week, I'm more connected to my body and spirit with a sense of calmness.

My friend Theresa, who is a yoga instructor and owner of Anahata Yoga and Healing Arts in Kingston, New York, says: "Yoga may not be able to fully replace hormones that are no longer being produced by a woman's body if due to surgery or menopause, but it can have a powerful effect on her state of mind as she learns to embrace her new body. Yoga's unique effect on the mind-body connection is one of the reasons it is routinely used to help overcome stress, depression, and other unpleasant emotional states. Even the simple act of stepping into our practice, and of committing to ourselves, sends self-love messages to the brain—and self-love is sometimes the most powerful medicine we can give ourselves."

Self-Love

Self-love was a powerful component of my healing. Most religions and spiritual traditions teach a version of the principles "Love they neighbor as thyself." It's the premise of showing the same kindness to others that we want to be shown to us. The problem is, we don't love ourselves enough, which adds to our stress levels.

During surgical menopause, we hate our symptoms and our bodies. But the last thing any of us needs is hate, especially when it comes to ourselves. Think of a child who falls and skins her knee. Her caregiver jumps in with gentle kindness and kisses the boo-boo to make it better. What if our symptoms are our bodies' ways of saying, "Hey? Love me. Hug me. Nurture me. Think good things about me. Get more rest. Stop feeding me that." Are we listening?

Self-love is the act of taking care of ourselves, which includes taking care of our bodies and health. Self-love is showing respect for ourselves and our well-being. Self-love is taking responsibility for our happiness. Self-love is accepting and embracing all the past, present, and future.

I love my body and all it's been through, even when it doesn't look or feel its best. I love the miracle that it can heal from the trauma of major surgery. I recognize that I woke up, I left the hospital, and I am making positive progress toward true health and balanced wellness every day. There are some aspects of my body, emotions, and life that I don't always like. I love myself anyway. I love my future self, the person I am becoming, and the woman right now who is lovable just because she exists. She is more than enough.

Forgiveness

There were times before and after surgery when I felt guilt and shame. I beat myself up with what I should have, could have, or shouldn't have done to prevent this thing called surgical menopause from happening. This only added to my stress. I chose to forgive myself. As I did this, I relaxed and allowed peace and harmony to be restored to my mind and heart. I tried not to feel bad for being emotional or for snapping at a loved one. At the same time, I learned to apologize often.

Meditation

Meditation was a tool that helped me create balance and reduce stress. The more my symptoms spun out of control, the more I required the silence that meditation brings. Meditation is a form of quiet listening and turning within.

The abruptness of losing our ovaries and uterus in surgery can destabilize our hormones and rob us of our sense of familiarity with our bodies. This can make us go through mood swings and affects our judgment. We may also grieve the loss of who we were. Healing our mind can work simultaneously and collaboratively with traditional medicine to help us put our lives and sense of selves back in order.

When my life gets hectic or symptoms spin out of control, I have discovered that I have a real choice: I can listen to the noise, focus on the symptoms, and pay attention to the minutia, or I can tune into the still small voice within me and listen for its guidance. I can learn to calm the chaos in my body and mind, which results in more peace and harmony in my life.

My meditation practice began with a daily fifteen-minute "sit." At first, the only goal was to keep my body still for the entire time. I'd often start out all bundled up, snuggled under a blanket. Halfway through, a hot flash would hit. I had two options.

1. Kick the blanket off, end my sit prematurely, and proceed to freak out.
2. Sit still and observe, allow the hot flash to come and go, and be unimpressed by it. I don't always get it right, but it has become an invaluable tool, nonetheless.

Meditation can also be practiced through making art or music, writing, coloring, and even gardening. Gardening is one of the few places where I lose all track of time. It's also the one place I'm not thinking of my next meal. Isn't it funny how something as simple as weeding the garden could bring peace, harmony, and weight loss?

When you think about how you plan to meditate, permit yourself to add any activity you do on your own where you go into the "zone" to the list. Meditation can be done seated, walking, or dancing. Look for places where you flow naturally and effortlessly in life.

CHAPTER 6

Thoughts, Words, and Feelings

WHEN I EXHAUSTED ALL the external resources of traditional and nontraditional routes to wellness along with lifestyle changes, I had nowhere to go but within. I am the only person in charge of my peace, joy, and bliss. And joy comes from within.

Why do I speak about joy? Because during my journey, there was darkness, sadness, and depression. As little girls, we read fairy tales about the prince riding in on a white horse to save us and living happily ever after. But the best satisfaction comes from you rescuing yourself. There is no need to give this power away. You are in charge of your joy. Don't give the responsibility to your child, parent, spouse, doctor, coworkers, boss, or anyone else.

In my experience with surgical menopause, I learned that I could control my feelings by changing my thoughts and words. This was a new concept to me. I had always been an emotional person, and I thought my emotions were strictly a result of my hormones and my external circumstances. When surgical menopause hit, my emotions became even more intense, especially those feelings of despair and sadness.

Before my surgery, when I was sad or emotional, Jim would ask, "What are you thinking right now in this moment?" He knew that my current feelings were a direct reflection of my current and past thoughts. His question brought me into the present moment, the only time when changes take place. I didn't get it right away. In fact, I rejected this theory for many years. It was easier to feel sorry for myself than it was to take responsibility. However, as I became more mindful of my thoughts and worked at keeping them more positive, my moods and emotions came into balance.

Anxiety and depression should not be taken lightly. Extreme conditions should be diagnosed and treated by medical professionals. However, I do believe that feelings are an indicator of our emotional wellness and can be a signal that something needs our attention. This is where we examine those spokes that I wrote about earlier. Let's take a closer, scientific look at the relationship between our thoughts and our feelings.

Science 101: Proteins, Peptides, and Feelings

Proteins are composed of amino acids linked together by peptide bonds. Our bodies use over 3,000 different proteins every day. Peptides are unique in that they are associated with every major emotion we experience.

There are uniquely shaped peptides emitted for each emotion and uniquely shaped receptors in all our cells that match these peptides. The peptides we emit the most have the most utilized receptors. And when cells reproduce, they develop more receptors for the emotions we use the most. The issue is that we lose receptors for the peptides we use the least.

Every eleven months, the body completely rebuilds itself with a new distribution of peptide receptors. Most cells reproduce themselves every twenty-one days.

The more receptors we have for a specific emotion, the greater the possibility that we can feel that emotion.

So, if we constantly and consistently allow and embrace emotions such as fear, guilt, shame, unworthiness, hurt feelings, anger, doubt, pity, overwhelm, sadness, depression, and confusion, then we will create more receptors for these emotions and have a greater capacity to feel these negative emotions.

By the same token, if we constantly and consistently allow and embrace feelings of gratitude, kindness, joy, love, serenity, passion, hope, inspiration, happiness, awe, and laughter, then we are literally creating ourselves to be more content.

Nobody else can live inside your skin or get into your head. You are the sculptor of your unique personal cellular structure, constantly making yourself over with your peptide receptors. Be sure to focus on the emotions you want to be able to feel the most intently and they will be the ones that replicate and get expressed more.

To increase the desired positive peptide production:

- Avoid saying negative statements out loud.
- Say positive statements out loud with intention.

As you develop habits through affirmations and changing your thoughts, words, and emotions, you will change your peptide receptors, and ultimately, change your life.

Our bodies are miracles, every day creating new cells and casting off new ones. Science has proven our entire bodies are replaced every few years. With this in mind, what are you building?

Thoughts

Our minds can be our most powerful tools or our worst enemies. A healthy life begins with a healthy mind. The connection between body, mind, and spirit is recognized by science.

Our negative thoughts and emotions are those of fear, anger, hatred, jealousy, and worry. Each of these increases our stress-related hormones, mainly cortisol, which has a negative effect on our health and specifically our menopause symptoms. If we let our thoughts go out of control, stress will most certainly manifest. When my thoughts get the best of me, the result shows up as a bad mood, sadness, or a panic attack.

When my system was compromised by the hormonal fluctuations of menopause, negative thoughts and emotions made my symptoms even more challenging. Positive thoughts and feelings of love, hope, and happiness helped to lessen my symptoms. The best part is, I can't have two masters. I am either negative or positive. I can't laugh and stay angry.

Our energy, feelings, thoughts, overall happiness, and success are truly within our control. But we must do our parts. We must consciously and consistently choose to be happy. To be grateful. To love. To forgive. To smile. This involves taking every thought captive, and choosing what we think about.

I spent over eight months reading the work of Charles Haanel, author of *The Master Key System*, published in 1912. Haanel writes: "Thought is a spiritual activity and is therefore creative. But make no mistake: Thought will create nothing unless it is consciously, systematically, and constructively directed; and herein is the difference between idle thinking, which is simply a dissipation of effort and constructive thinking, which means practically unlimited achievement."[8] If our thoughts directly affect our experiences, interactions, and lives, then we have the power to change our world and the world around us by changing our thoughts.

But what if you have bad thoughts or "stinkin' thinkin'"? Perhaps cynics and negativity surround you. This can certainly create a toxic mind. Regardless of what you've experienced, learned, and created as a habit, you have the power to replace bad thoughts with good. Good thoughts create good habits, which create changes in our inner and outer worlds.

I believe my body can heal through thoughts, prayer, and meditation, however, that doesn't mean that I am saying that if I'm good enough, bad things won't happen or that if I can heal myself then perhaps I also caused the condition that led to the need for surgery. I am suggesting that pain, illness, disease, and surgery can be a wake-up call. It's a signal that a spoke or two in the wheel of my well-being bicycle may be broken and it's time to address them and get back in balance.

Tools to Change Your Thoughts
Adjust Your Attitude

As I mentioned earlier, I use BHRT to manage my symptoms. Once a month, I stop using it per my doctor's instructions. When my symptoms reappear, mainly hot flashes and night sweats, I start again. There are times where my menopausal symptoms are worse than others. Feeling sorry for myself doesn't help me. Instead of continuing down a road of complaining, whining, and blaming, I start praising and counting my blessings. I commit myself to an attitude of gratitude and I transform my world.

What am I grateful for in this moment? What do I want to remember? The benefits of gratitude are highest when I express it daily in writing. Every day I write down three new things that I am grateful for. In the past, I've done this in a journal and reviewed it often. I've also written them on a stack of index cards, so I can flash through them several times a day. I include wonderful things that I observed or experienced in the past twenty-four hours. As I focus on the positive, how I perceive the world around me changes.

Here are some grateful thoughts that you could practice

thinking or say out loud to get started. Invent more.

- "Thank you for my legs; they get me where I want to go."
- "Thank you for my eyes and the ability to see the beauty of the world."
- "Thank you for my heart that beats without any input on my part and has the capacity to love deeply."
- "Thank you for this hot flash; it allows me to be present in my body and aware of my surroundings."
- "Thank you for an amazing love."
- "Thank you for family and friendships."
- "Thank you for my home, a working vehicle, and indoor plumbing."
- "Thank you for the ability to earn money, give regularly, and save."

Attitude combined with the right perspective reminds us to be grateful and live in the solution, instead of staying stuck in our problems. When I fight with a loved one, I remember that my friend Lauren's brother literally fought for his life after a motorcycle accident that ultimately would take his arm and leg. *I am grateful for my limbs.*

When I struggle with hot flashes, night sweats, insomnia, brain fog, or other menopausal symptoms, I remember that my friend Jackie lost her fifteen-year-old daughter to cancer. *I am grateful for my life.*

While I was writing this book, my cousin Kim lost her battle with brain cancer. Her husband, son, mom, sister, family, and friends would all give just about anything to have one more day with her. We don't have to lose a loved one to appreciate life. A simple way to feel more gratitude is to read an obituary daily and ask yourself, "What would this person give to have one more day?" My point is, we don't have to stop living until our condition has resolved. We can simply be unimpressed by it.

There is a story in the Bible about the apostle Paul and the thorn in his flesh. It doesn't say if it was physical. We just know Paul saw it as a form of pain. Paul asked God three times to remove the thorn and was denied, learning grace and strength in the process.

Don't we do the same? We think we could be more effective or productive without an ailment or symptom. We wait until we feel good before we step into our purpose or passion or greatness. What if the goal is to live with joy despite our challenges? Despite surgical menopause? What if we are to live on purpose despite the thorns in our lives and how they manifest for us? Everybody has experienced a thorn in her side at some point. The question is, what is your attitude toward your thorn?

Get a New Perspective

I am technically postmenopausal; however, I do still have symptoms that may continue for months or years to come. It helps me to remember that no matter how bad my symptoms get they will not kill me. They are just uncomfortable. It is up to me to learn to live in balance, health, harmony, and freedom. It is up to me to control and empower myself, so I remain the healthy, joyful woman I know myself to be. When I do this, I find myself with a whole new outlook. My symptoms may not change, my perspective does.

The first year after surgery, one of the surgical menopause symptoms that plagued me was a loss of libido, which had an unfortunate impact on my sex life. However, when I went off BHRT, suddenly I was dealing with vaginal dryness and atrophy, which for me, was much worse. And more painful. Pain can be a strong motivator. Suddenly, I wanted to have sex. More than anything. My libido was in fact strong. And I raced back to my doctor who gave me a beautiful little lotion I could apply daily to resolve the physical issues. The BHRT I went on made my vagina young again. This physical challenge put things into perspective for me. I discovered that my libido didn't have to be a physical or psychological issue. It could be a mindset. I could change my mind about wanting to have sex.

Another perspective to examine is our beliefs around menopause and aging. As women, we fear being sidelined from the mainstream of life, put out to pasture. Yet there are so many tremendous examples of women in midlife and beyond who are doing remarkable things. They are writing books, rescuing children, serving in the Senate and House of Representatives, and inspiring future generations. They are purposeful and contribute so much value to their families and communities. We can too.

Change Your Focus

Did you ever notice that what you think about grows and what you forget about atrophies? Do a mental check-in. Are you focused on every menopause symptom? In general, do you focus on your problems or blessings?

I'm the queen of research. Surgical menopause was all I talked about and thought about for too long. I spent over eighteen months looking for answers. Until I let go. I fired Dr. Google. I stopped searching and researching. I got quiet. I went within. I accepted that I might never get rid of my symptoms and I learned that I could manage them to the best of my ability.

As a kid growing up, my dad taught me how to ride a bike and drive a car. He taught me not to look at the mailboxes along the side of the road because where my gaze went, the car followed. Focusing on my body works the same way. When I focus on hot flashes, I seem to get more hot flashes. As I focused on being healthy and strong, living a life of laughter and harmony, my symptoms subsided. Balance, freedom, and joy arrive.

There is an old saying "I'll believe it when I see it." The reality is, you must believe it before you can see it. Focus on the parts of you that are healthy. Your lungs are working. Your heart is beating. Your feet and legs are holding you up. Change your focus to what is right in your life and you'll feel much better.

Guard What Comes In

In today's world, we are inundated with music, movies, newspapers, social media, texts from our friends, and television programming. This is an area we can choose what we allow in to be positive or negative.

When Jim and I started dating, he would ask what movie I wanted to see. I always picked the drama. He always picked the comedy. He still does. The dramas were my way of leaning into sadness, darkness, and negative emotions. The comedy was his way of lightening things up and adding more laughter to our lives.

After my surgery, I realized how much I needed comedy to heal me and help me unwind. I took an inventory of what I was listening to, watching, and reading. I made sure I had a balance or overflow of things and people that lifted me up, changed my mood for the better or empowered me.

At this juncture in my life where recovery and stabilization of my health was a significant goal, I also benefited from doing an inventory of relationships.

We all know toxic people who spew negativity everywhere they go. When we are feeling challenged, it is a good idea to surround ourselves with people who lift us up and inspire. When we are feeling our best, we can share our positivity with those who could use our light and love.

Swap It

Have you ever tried to release something from your thoughts, but the more you focus on releasing it, the more you think about it? It's like me telling you not to think about a talking rabbit and all you do is think about Bugs Bunny. We can't stop thinking about something. Nor can we think about two things at once. We must substitute one thing for another.

We can choose what we think about. So, make a list of fond memories or pleasant thoughts to have on hand. Then, if your thoughts and feelings start to stray toward the negative, you can quickly swap them with something positive, funny, or beautiful. The goal is to avoid thinking any negative thoughts, as well as release all complaining, blaming, or whining.

When I catch myself thinking negatively, I allow myself seven seconds to turn the negative thought into a positive. I learned to swap thoughts of self-pity for thoughts of warm, sunny days at the beach.

Words

Our words reinforce our thoughts and add fuel to our feelings. There were ancient societies, including those of the ancient Greeks and Romans, whose members believed that what is said out loud is called into existence. When my menopausal symptoms were at their worst, I examined my language to become more aware of what I was speaking into existence. Was I speaking about myself as a woman who was limited and suffering or empowered and healthy?

Have you ever said something like "I look fat. I'm ugly. I'm getting old. I'm not enough. I'm stupid. I'm always wrong"? When we do this, we are using words against ourselves.

To be empowered and healthy women, we must learn to be impeccable with our words and say only positive things that build us up. Try saying "I love you" out loud to yourself daily.

This is an incredibly powerful phrase, especially if done while looking at yourself in the mirror.

Tools to Change Your Language

Change Your Story

Do you relive your trauma or celebrate your victories? Do you call all your friends to tell your story again and again? If you are sharing your victories, congratulations. Keep sharing. If you are sharing trauma, perhaps it's time to let your sad stories go.

One day when I was complaining about surgical menopause, my friend said, "I'm sorry you needed surgery. Now tell me about the veggies in your garden or the last big laugh you had." With this request, my friend showed compassion *and* helped me to focus on the positive and change the story I had been repeating to anyone that would listen.

Jim and I have a three times rule: If you hear yourself say something three times, make sure you are listening. As soon as we've complained about something three times in a row, it's time to recognize and do something about it. At the minimum, we stop saying the negative and stop leaning into it. When we catch ourselves saying "I'm tired" for the third time in a week, we either make a point to catch up on sleep or we change our language. We say, "I'm vibrant. I'm alive. I have all the energy I require." We begin to take steps to change the state of our being. This doesn't mean life necessarily gets easy; it means we do life with ease. We let go of struggle and focus on solutions, not obstacles, symptoms, or problems.

Not everyone will want to do the work I'm suggesting in these pages. It is common to want to take a pill, use cream, or meet a prince to make all our problems go away. There are times I did. And still do. But to come back strong and find balanced wellness after surgical menopause, I decided that I could rewrite my own story and make it one filled with positive celebrations and victories.

Speak It into Existence

There are subtleties in language that affect our thoughts and feelings and beliefs about who we are. For example, we can start sentences with "I want to be" or with "I am." Imagine if all day long I said or thought "I want to be healthy." The word *want* signals to my brain that I have a need because I don't yet have something. When I change "I want" to "I am," and affirm it in word and thought all day long, I send signals to my brain that I already am what I want to become.

Here are a few phrases I have learned to change to speak it into existence.

- I want to feel young and vibrant. *I am young and vibrant.*
- I want to be healthy. *I am healthy.*
- I want to be strong and well balanced. *I am strong and well balanced.*
- I want love. *I am love. I am loved.*

Express Joy

I love listening to Ryan Seacrest on the radio when he encourages listeners, "Tell me something good." It reinforces the idea that joy should be shared and celebrated together.

The secret to abundant joy is in the expression of it. As a child, I had no problem living in my curiosity and expressing my sheer delight at what I found. I also had no problem expressing my discontent without a filter. At some point, I learned that anger and negative emotions were not acceptable in all circles, so I begin to stuff these feelings. The problem was, the more I stuffed the negative, the bigger the habit of suppression I formed. Soon I was stuffing joy as well as pain.

Affirm It

Affirmations are positive, specific statements that can help reprogram our minds and create better thought habits. They are stated in the present tense and can literally change the blueprint of how we think. This is not a fake-it-until-you-make-it mentality, but more of a fake-it-until-you-feel-it or fake-it-until-you-become-it mentality.

My favorite affirmation, which I say many times each day, is from Charles Haanel: "I am whole, perfect, strong, powerful, loving, harmonious, and happy."

Affirmations work best when written down and spoken out loud. I advocate writing them down over and over every day. There's something about connecting the muscle memory of writing to the brain that is especially powerful. Here are a few of my daily affirmations.

- I have true health in body, mind, spirit, and emotion.
- My life is in balance with work, play, and rest.
- I sleep easily and soundly and wake up vibrant and joyful.
- I laugh with ease.
- It feels wonderful to relax, rest, and play.

Here are some additional affirmations you may wish to explore. Take what you need and create your own.

- I allow life to flow through me.
- I love and approve of myself.
- As I release the past, the new and vital enter.
- Letting go is easy.
- I trust my inner voice.
- I bring peace to every corner of my life.
- I think and speak only words of love.
- I approve of myself.
- I am balanced.
- I am peaceful through all changes.
- Bodily processes are normal and natural.

- I accept my body.
- I am healthy.
- I am creative, productive, and purposeful.
- I release all anger and resentment.
- I accept all good things without guilt.
- I hear and live the truth of my heart.

Feelings

Feelings are a great indicator of what we are thinking. When we take a thought, and add feeling and emotion to it, we build a powerful force of desire, motivation, and action. During my recovery from surgical menopause, I learned to release and express my feelings. Some days this involves celebrating joy. Other days, it means I allow myself a good cry or a long nap.

Menopause brought feelings of sadness, anger, loss, and overwhelm. At times, I felt "less than" and not good enough. When I feel something negative, I examine what I *feel* versus what I *know*. I can't always trust how I feel. I can feel alone and not be alone. I can feel fat and not be fat. I can feel weak and pitiful, and yet know that I am strong and empowered.

After surgery, I wept about things that didn't normally make me cry, like shells in my scrambled eggs, broken pencil leads, or Jim telling me he loved me. Eventually, I recognized that these emotions weren't based on my beliefs or desires or fears. They were a sign of my body being unbalanced. I learned to observe the outbursts with curiosity and detachment, rather than "owning" them.

Over time, I learned to release the sad and angry feelings with a breath, laugh, scream, punch, or sometimes even a kick. (Hopefully at something that was soft and indestructible.) Other times release came through tears, sex, or exercise.

Tools to Change Your Emotions

In my journey of healing through surgical menopause, I learned that I could take control of my emotions by changing my thoughts and words. This came with the decision to be happy before I felt it. When I choose to be happy, then I am literally one smile, laugh, or dance move away from changing my emotions.

Celebrate Victories and Strengths

Two tools that helped me restore a positive attitude and encourage myself when menopause symptoms were at their worst were a kudos box and flashcards.

Kudos are praise and honor received for an achievement. Over the years, I have saved greeting cards, notes, and awards that encouraged me or celebrated my victories. I keep them all in a kudos shoebox and when I'm feeling sad, I sift through them and find my spirit lifted. I also set up a kudos folder in my email and anytime I receive an email that thanked me or acknowledged my strengths, I file it away for a rainy day.

I also utilize flash cards to increase my confidence and positive outlook. Remember when we were kids and our parents or teachers used flashcards to help us learn math or the names of colors and animals? You can create flashcards out of index cards. Start with writing out twenty achievements you are proud of, one per card. An achievement could be that you graduated from high school or you made your bed this morning. Add to your flash cards daily things you love about yourself and past victories. Examples can include you woke up from surgery, learned to meditate, started exercising again, or any other step toward healing from surgical menopause you took or accomplished.

Flash through your cards daily. Do it when you first wake up, before you go to bed, after every meal, and whenever you start to feel sad. As you focus on your strengths and the positive, you'll feel your mood lightened and lifted.

Smile

Our feelings are also contagious. One day, I noticed that every person I encountered smiled at me like I was their best friend and said hello. I thought, Wow! Everyone is so friendly today. It was like everyone was in a good mood. Then I realized it was me that was in a good mood. I was smiling. I was calm, relaxed, and walking with confidence. I was greeting everyone like they were my best friend. My smile was contagious, as were my positive feelings.

Laugh

Q: How do you catch a RARE rabbit?
    A: Easy. U-NIQUE up on him.
    Q: How do you catch a TAME rabbit?
    A: TAME way, silly.

Would you believe that this is my favorite joke? Just in trying to tell it, I get the giggles. I don't know why. It tickles my funny bone. People look at me like I'm crazy or ridiculous, but after a while they can't help but join me. Laughter is a strong antidote for a bad mood. Laughter releases negativity in its path. It's hard to be sad or angry when we're laughing.

As part of a conscious plan to fill my mind and heart with all things of love, laughter, and fun, I record (showing my age here, as technically now I am DVR-ing) daily episodes of *The Ellen Show*. I bought DVDs of *I Love Lucy* and *The Carol Burnett Show*. I subscribed on YouTube to Jimmy Fallon and Carpool Karaoke. When Jim asks me to go to the movies, I pick a comedy. As I focus on laughter, I feel better. I'm not suggesting that I won't ever watch another serious or dramatic movie. I'm saying that when my health, body, or emotions are compromised, as they were with surgical menopause, it's best for me to choose to fill life with positive and funny moments through movies, televisions, and books, or happy and inspiring posts on Pinterest and Instagram.

Sing, Shout, Jump, or Dance

Another way to change our negative feelings or energy is through singing, shouting, jumping, or dancing. One morning I thought I was home alone. I grabbed my iPhone and blared Nickelback while I danced, jumped, and bounced around the living room. I was energized and invigorated. I was truly dancing as if no one was watching because no one was. Until that is, Jim came around the corner. I'm not sure who was more surprised!

Jim smiled with joy. I believed because I was dancing with glee and wild abandon.

Then again, it could have been because I was naked.

Either way, it was a great way to start the day and a powerful lesson in being able to affect my feelings and emotions, as well as those of the people around me by simple movement.

Get Dressed

Sometimes all I need to do to get out of a valley of darkness is to take a shower. Simply getting out of my pajamas can improve my mood. I put on clean clothes, brush my hair, and add some make-up and jewelry. Clothing can cheer us up. The right outfit can reflect a mood or change it. It can reflect pride and pleasure.

Strike a Pose

Whether you choose a victory pose with arms up in the air in the shape of a V, or a Wonder Woman pose with hands on hips, practicing this activity for as little as two minutes every day can train your brain that you are victorious and powerful. You are whole, perfect, strong, powerful, loving, harmonious, and happy. And that can improve any gal's mood in an instant.

CHAPTER 7

Come Back Strong

THE FOUR MONTHS BEFORE my surgery and twenty months after were the darkest period of my life. Surgical menopause rattled my cage and threatened to rob me of my confidence, sexuality, and motivation. And I'm no stranger to pain; I survived child molestation, an abusive relationship, divorce, and watched loved ones deal with disease. However, it was in the journey through the darkness that I discovered my purpose, deeper passions, and ultimately, joy. It was where I was forced to examine the spokes on my wellness wheel, so I could reclaim and maintain my balance. It was where I learned that setbacks are setups for comebacks.

Choices

Every one of us has a choice to follow faith or fear. We can fear the worst, thinking we are never going to be the same or get well, or we can have faith that every single day we are being healed, restored, and will come back stronger than ever. We can have faith that we're not growing older; we're growing more youthful, better, wiser, calmer, leaner, and stronger.

Have hope. You will get through this. BHRT and other nat-ural solutions can help. But some symptoms will require hard work, a positive mental attitude, and patience. It may feel dark where you are, but light and joy will come again.

Part of faith comes with a decision. You decide today to be strong and believe that your current condition won't beat you. You decide to look at alternative solutions. You decide to find joy right where you are and trust that happiness will follow.

You don't have to be a victim of your circumstances. Two men grow up with abusive fathers. One continues the legacy of anger, jealousy, insecurity, and bullying. One breaks the pat-tern and focuses on love, always wears a smile, is confident and trusting. Same history, same experience, same circum-stance, different outcome. And different impact on the world. The difference is how these two men chose to live their lives and whom they chose to become.

The same can happen with us. Two women. Both are thrust into sudden surgical menopause. One leans in, gains weight, and grows more and more withdrawn, melancholy, and de-feated. The other woman does everything in her power to heal, live her passion, find her purpose, and lead a life of love, laughter, and freedom. Same experience, same circumstance, different outcome. And different impact on the world.

Discover Your Purpose

In my research on the symptoms of menopause, I heard from women who complained of a lack of drive or motivation. I could relate. At the time, I thought this was a new symptom related to menopause. Now, looking back with more perspec-tive, I realize it was something I had struggled with for many years. Menopause heightened my sense of longing for purpose.

Don't get me wrong, I live a beautiful life. However, in the past, there was always this angst, this unrest, this questioning, this . . . searching. Menopause brought it up for examination. I began to reflect on my past with a strong desire to heal areas of stress and trauma and confusion. I also began to look to my future and ponder who I wanted to be.

Who knew that all along what I was searching for was me, Lori. I was searching and waiting for myself to wake up, show up, take responsibility, and be the hero in my own life. And in becoming the hero, I found purpose. I found clarity. Knowing I could help others through their recovery has given me the drive to push myself to do more.

When your life has purpose, you have unlimited energy and joy. Psychologist Shawn Achor, one of the world's leading experts on the connection between happiness and success, defines happiness as the "joy you feel moving toward your potential."[9]

Think of your purpose as a present, as in a gift. Ask yourself, "Am I withholding myself or my gifts from the world? Am I living small? Or am I sharing myself, my gifts, my talents, and my message with those around me? Am I shining my light so brightly that I give others permission to shine theirs?"

Each one of us was born with gifts to share with the world, even if we don't always know what they are. We can discover them at any time. About eighteen months after surgery, I began writing my purpose statement. This was where an awakening happened and I discovered my true passion and purpose as a writer. I started the statement with 400 words and then narrowed it down to one sentence.

I am a best-selling author inspiring people to live a life of true health, love, laughter, and freedom through my writing, speaking, and coaching.

In the beginning, I didn't have a lot of confidence. This was a bold statement for someone who had only published in a magazine and on the web. But to this day, as I read this statement out loud, I *feel* it. I feel the presence of it, which shows up in the way I present myself to the world while presenting my gifts of courage, enthusiasm, persistence, passion, and authenticity to it. Who am I not to step into this purpose and become all that I was created to be?

In hindsight, my purpose was with me all along. *True health* showed up in many areas of my life. I've been an athlete all my life. I have a bachelor's degree in recreation. I became a wellness coach and a sports nutritionist because I have always strived to live the healthiest life possible. It's in my blood.

Love and *laughter* are also two constants in my life. I love deeply and I laugh often. I'm grateful to have found a partner who holds love and laughter as great values in his life. I believe everyone deserves to feel love and laugh daily. And it is our responsibility to share it wherever we go.

I discovered that autonomy is a pivotal need for me personally. Autonomy can be defined as self-governance or *freedom* from external control or influence, as independence. Two of my favorite words are wrapped up in this definition: *freedom* and *independence.*

This may make you laugh, but when I turned eighteen and registered to vote, I registered as an independent because I liked the word. Independent was what I wanted to be. Years later, as I left an abusive relationship, it was *freedom* I was seeking, and ironically, it came right around Independence Day, my favorite holiday. What I wanted at so many crossroads of my life was *freedom.* I wanted freedom in my body, freedom in my food, and freedom from suppression and feelings of guilt and shame. I wanted the freedom to be me. Unapologetic. Unashamed. Real. Raw. Me.

Another interesting fact? I'm an independent associate of a billion-dollar wellness company whose mission is to: "To impact world health and free people from physical and financial pain." Again, it points me right to *true health* and *freedom.*

As true health, love, laughter, and freedom rose in me, I discovered that I not only wanted these things for myself, I wanted to inspire others to have them as well. Once I discovered the *why*, the *how* became crystal clear: through my writing, speaking, and coaching.

Discovering our purposes can be scary. We may have mindsets like Peter's on the Sea of Galilee. His fears kept him in the boat, instead of stepping out on the water where Jesus was. We may stay "in the boat" too, not necessarily because it's comfortable but because it's familiar. At the same time, our hearts yearn for something more. Something great. We long to lead lives of passion and purpose. We long to "walk on water."

I believe I have a unique purpose and ability to help others. As I worked through the healing process in my own life, I have learned that I have solutions to offer other women facing surgery or experiencing surgical menopause. To help, I don't have to wait until I figure it all out. As I help others, I advance my healing.

Uncover and Embrace Your Passion

You may not know or realize your purpose right away. You can discover it by following your passion and living in your curiosity. During surgical menopause, you may discover, like me, that you are not passionate about your job. Maybe you never were. You may not be able to change that right now. What's a girl to do? You can focus on all the positives . . . the hours, the proximity, the benefits, maybe merely that you earn a paycheck. And then you can pour your passion into other areas of your life outside of work, whether it's through sports or fitness, art, music, dance, service, or philanthropy. Choose to focus on what you can change, and accept what you cannot.

For me, one of the places I'm most happy is on my bike. Cycling was something I loved as a child and then detoured away from in my late teens and twenties. Rediscovering this passion in my thirties was like a rebirth. Just like when I was a kid, I love riding my bike. I love sprinting, pace lines, climbing up hills, flying down hills, seeing new places, traveling further than I could on two feet, pushing my body, and feeling both exhilarated and exhausted. Riding my bike in beautiful places is my heart's desire, and I get to do it with my best friend, Jim. Regardless of the circumstances of my life or even my menopausal symptoms, if I can ride, then life is good.

So often, we stop dreaming. We forget our first loves. We give up on our passions. It could be due to time or money. It could be because life became about the struggle instead of the dream. It's time you gave yourself permission to dream. What was your passion as a child? Are you still doing it? If you don't know what it is, get quiet. Your mind, body, spirit, and emotion are connected internally and universally. We can't hear the still small voice pointing us in the right direction if we're busy, tense, or stressed.

Spend at least fifteen minutes daily and in prayer or meditation. Buy a journal and write daily. Explore your past and remember points in your life you were most happy. What were you doing? Were you riding your bike? Gardening? Singing? Teaching? Working with your hands? *Are you still doing it?* If not, consider finding ways to bring it back into your life. My friend Wendy loved to sing and act through high school and college. She got married, had kids, and somewhere along the line stopped singing. Menopause caused her to reevaluate her life and in the process, rediscover her passion. She found a local theater and now enjoys singing and acting there on a regular basis.

My friend Sierra is a runner. She has competed at the professional level in marathons and triathlons. During menopause, she found purpose in coaching her son's cross-country running team, while continuing to indulge her own passion for running.

The Next Chapter

What if surgical menopause is just what you need to turn the page and bring you to the next chapter of your life, where the real work begins, where you start really living?

Menopause can take a decade and can be a time of indecision, emotional turmoil, and frustration. Surgical menopause pushed me through at a much faster pace. Peace, harmony, joy, and purpose were waiting for me on the other side. My symptoms have not gone away completely, but I'm able to manage them better through the tools and practices discussed in this book.

Surgery led me to a life of service, inspiration, and love. It's where I gave myself permission to live a pain-free and productive life. It's where I learned self-love, forgiveness, and grace. I've grown more comfortable in my skin through this experience. I recognized my priorities and I became more interested in things like joy and freedom. I became more open to living my truth and listening to my heart. I no longer feel the need to ask for permission or to offer explanations. I don't justify or defend. I live, love, and laugh. I am free.

For a long time, I was a great pretender. I pretended I didn't know what the next chapter was or the next step. But in my heart, I truly *did* know what to do next. The answer terrified me.

What are you pretending you don't know? What are you afraid of? Is it that the next step is to quit your job? Write a book? Leave your spouse? Go back to school? Start a charity? Go on a mission trip? Call someone you haven't spoken to in a long time? Forgive? Ask for forgiveness? Love someone that is acting unlovable? Adopt? Give more? Any of these steps can leave a woman filled with fear, but there is no difference between something that scares us and something that excites us. To our bodies and minds, it's the same exact thing.

A Time for All Things

Surgical menopause may be different for every woman, depending on her age, personal medical history, family medical history, stress levels, mindset, and lifestyle choices, including exercise and nutrition. There may be times you cry and times you laugh, times you rest and times you dance, times you heal and times you grieve. And a time when you rise. Finding balanced wellness after surgical menopause will take time and patience. Go within. Learn what you want. Figure out what you need. And come back strong.

Questions You May Wish to Ask Your Doctor

AS YOU PREPARE FOR surgery and your initial recovery, you may or may not have questions. Looking back, I thought I was prepared. However, I had not educated myself on what comes after hysterectomy and oophorectomy: surgical menopause. The following is a list of questions you can print out and take with you to your doctor.

- Is this surgery necessary? Are there other options?
- Will decisions need to be made while I'm unconscious?
- Are there any nonsurgical options I could try before agreeing to surgery?
- Are there benefits, or risks, involved with doing nothing and continuing to monitor my situation.
- When you say full hysterectomy, what exactly will you be removing?
- Are there any organs worth fighting for?
- What are the repercussions of life without a uterus, ovaries, and cervix?

- Are there any further risks for me post hysterectomy and oophorectomy? Are there benefits?
- What can I do ahead of time to prepare well for surgery and surgical menopause?
- May I use arnica, bromelain, or peppermint tablets before and after surgery to speed healing?
- What will my sex life be like after surgery? Will I still enjoy sex? Will orgasms be the same, harder, or better?
- Will sex be painful? For how long?
- Will my vagina be shorter?
- Are there support groups or books you can recommend?
- What does my partner need to know/prepare for?
- I have small children. What tasks will I be too limited to do?
- What can I expect for recovery time?
- What scars will I have?
- Will I require hormone replacement therapy? How soon will I start it after surgery?
- How long will I take hormones?
- Is taking hormones safe for me?
- Can you help me understand the difference between bi-oidentical hormone replacement therapy (BHRT) and hormone replacement therapy (HRT)? Which type do you recommend for me—and why?
- What symptoms can I reasonably expect hormone therapy to eliminate?
- How long should I wait before starting or changing the dosage of hormones?
- What symptoms can I affect through lifestyle changes?
- How long will my symptoms last?
- Does your practice offer counseling or emotional support?
- What type of follow-up will be required and recommended?

Notes

1. Suzanne Somers, *The Sexy Years: Discover the Hormone Connection: The Secret to Fabulous Sex, Great Health, and Vitality, for Women and Men* (New York: Three Rivers Press, 2004), p. 2.
2. Camille Lawson, "Hormones: The Key to Vibrant Health and Sexuality for Women," *FemMED®, Intrinsic Supplements for Women,* (accessed October 13, 2017), http://femmed.com/hormones-the-key-to-vibrant-health-and-sexuality-for-women-part-one.
3. Don Miguel Ruiz, *The Four Agreements: A Practical Guide to Personal Freedom* (San Rafael, CA.: Amber-Allen Publishing, 1997), pp. 28–29.
4. Josh Axe, "Top 15 Anti-Inflammatory Foods," *Dr. Axe Food Is Medi*cine, (accessed October 13, 2017), https://draxe.com/anti-inflammatory-foods.
5. Sharon Feiereisen, "25 Best Foods for Menopause," *Eat This, Not That* (accessed September 7, 2016), http://www.eatthis.com/menopause.
6. Josh Axe, "8 Natural Remedies for Menopause Relief," *Dr. Axe Food Is Medicine,* (accessed October 13, 2017), https://draxe.com/5-natural-remedies-menopause-relief.
7. "Five Foods and Drinks to Avoid during Menopause," *34 Menopause Symptoms* (accessed October 13, 2017), https://www.34-menopause-symptoms.com/articles/5-foods-and-drinks-to-stay-away-from-during-menopause.htm.
8. Charles F. Haanel, "Part Thirteen," *The Master Key System: Your Step-by-Step Guide to Using the Law of Attraction* (New York: Jeremy P. Tarcher, 2007), pp. 145–156. Originally published as a correspondence course in 1912, and then as a book in 1917.

9. Shawn Achor (accessed October 23, 2017), http://www. shawnachor.com.

Resources

Lori is available for personal one-on-one coaching in weight loss, energy, performance, healthy aging, and wealth creation. Her professional guidance and experience in each of these areas will assist you to create results and success in your own life.

Join her on these social networks.
- Facebook: www.facebook.com/LoriKingCycleChick
- Twitter: www.twitter.com/LoriCycleChick
- LinkedIn: www.linkedin.com/in/Lori-Ann-King
- Instagram: www.instagram.com/LoriKingCycleChick
- YouTube: www.youtube.com/c/LoriKingWellness

Hire her as a speaker on topics such as:
- Exercise, Nutrition, and Hormones, Oh My!
- Life Lessons from the Bike
- Balanced Wellness Through Menopause

For more information, please visit her website:
www.LoriAnnKing.com

Join her mailing list at: www.loriannking.com/opt-in

Download her free reports:
- *Lori's Food Plan for Stubborn Weight Loss*
- *10 Simple Tips for Balanced Wellness and Healthy Living*
- *Questions to Ask Your Doctor Before Surgery*

Index

About the Author

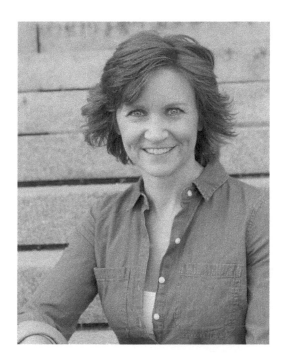

LORI ANN KING is a writer, speaker, blogger, certified sports nutritionist, and wellness coach with over eight years of experience in health and wellness.

Lori is also a cyclist and body builder, and was a runner for over twenty-five years, competing in races ranging in length from two to 26.2 miles. She has an undergraduate degree in Recreation from Western State College of Colorado and an advanced certificate in Information Management from Syracuse University.

Lori currently resides in the Hudson Valley of New York with her husband, Jim.

Lightning Source UK Ltd.
Milton Keynes UK
UKHW01f1628300918
329774UK00010B/168/P